U0188692

馆史钩沉
图说上海中医药博物馆

主编·李赣　副主编·全瑾　绘画·罗希贤 董林祥

汉英对照 Chinese-English Version

An Illustrated History of the Shanghai Museum of Traditional Chinese Medicine

Editor-in-Chief · Li Gan　Associate Editor · Quan Jin　Illustrators · Luo Xixian Dong Linxiang

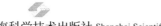
上海科学技术出版社 Shanghai Scientific & Technical Publishers

图书在版编目（ＣＩＰ）数据

馆史钩沉 ： 图说上海中医药博物馆 ： 汉英对照 /
李赣主编. -- 上海 ： 上海科学技术出版社，2023.11
ISBN 978-7-5478-6394-7

Ⅰ．①馆… Ⅱ．①李… Ⅲ．①中国医药学－医学史－
博物馆－上海－图解 Ⅳ．①R-092

中国国家版本馆CIP数据核字(2023)第207455号

馆史钩沉——图说上海中医药博物馆（汉英对照）

主　编　李　赣
副主编　仝　瑾
绘　画　罗希贤　董林祥

上海世纪出版（集团）有限公司
上海科学技术出版社　出版、发行
（上海市闵行区号景路159弄A座9F-10F）
邮政编码201101　www.sstp.cn
苏州工业园区美柯乐制版印务有限责任公司印刷
开本　787×1092　1/16　印张　7.5
字数　90千字
2023年11月第1版　2023年11月第1次印刷
ISBN 978-7-5478-6394-7 / R·2875
定价：98.00元

本书如有缺页、错装或坏损等严重质量问题，请向印刷厂联系调换

内容提要

Summary

1938 年 7 月，中国最早的医学史博物馆——中华医学会医史博物馆创建，创办人是中国著名医史学家王吉民先生。博物馆的诞生是以中国学者为代表的中国人民爱国自强的产物。

本书以中国传统连环画的方式，勾勒出上海中医药博物馆 / 中华医学会医史博物馆的创立、发展脉络，展示博物馆 80 多年的发展探索和取得的成绩。

In July 1938, the Museum of Medical History of the Chinese Medical Association, the first medical history museum in China, was established. The museum emerged from the patriotic and self-strengthening efforts of the Chinese people, represented by Chinese scholars like its founder, Mr. Wang Jimin, a renowned medical historian.

This book depicts how the museum was established and developed through comic strips rich in traditional Chinese elements. It showcases the museum's achievements spanning 80 years of exploration and advancement.

编委会名单

Editor's List

主编 · 李　赣

副主编 · 全　瑾

编写人员 · （按姓氏笔画排序）

全　瑾　陈侣华　李　赣　罗月琴　郑　芬
俞宝英　韩　俊　燕竞飞　濮姗姗

绘画 · 罗希贤　董林祥

译员 · （按姓氏笔画排序）

刘萍萍　阮子蓉　张晓晨　陈南雄　林　淼
周　恩　浦文怡　董尧琦　覃健强　赖碧怡
薛玲玲

Editor-in-Chief

Li Gan

Associate Editor

Quan Jin

Editors (In the order of surname strokes)

Quan Jin　　Chen Lyuhua　　Li Gan　　Luo Yueqin　　Zheng Fen
Yu Baoying　　Han Jun　　Yan Jingfei　　Pu Shanshan

Illustrators

Luo Xixian　　Dong Linxiang

Translators (In the order of surname strokes)

Liu Pingping　　Ruan Zirong　　Zhang Xiaochen　　Chen Nanxiong　　Lin Miao
Zhou En　　Pu Wenyi　　Dong Yaoqi　　Qin Jianqiang　　Lai Biyi
Xue Lingling

编写说明

池浜开馆露初容，三徙张江智创城。里外杏荫观杏展，万千文物透春风。1938 年 7 月，上海池浜路 41 号，中国第一家医学史博物馆—中华医学会医史博物馆诞生了，创办人是中国著名医史学家王吉民先生。博物馆的创立在旧中国起到了唤醒民族觉悟和振奋爱国情怀的作用，它是以中国学者为代表的中国人民爱国自强的产物，是一个国家、一个民族的历史文化面貌与精神灵魂的生动体现。

历史的脚步清晰凝重，文化的传承绵延不息。博物馆的建立，不仅在中医药文物的收藏保护方面有着重要的意义，而且在医学教育、文化教育、爱国主义教育、科学知识普及等方面起着积极作用。如今，博物馆已走过 80 多年的发展历程。抚今追昔，博物馆经历了不同时期的馆址变迁、馆名变更，历经八十载风雨砥砺，有创业中的举步维艰，有奋进中的探索思考，有喜悦中的跨越发展。回眸昨日，枝叶繁茂，基石稳固，未来更美。

八秩奋斗，续写华章。本书通过一幅幅图片、一幕幕往事，回顾了博物馆 80 年的发展探索和取得的成绩。不由引起我们对过去岁月的思念，对我们先辈们的崇敬，更为我们拥有中医药这一伟大的医药文化瑰宝而自豪。经过一代代博物馆人的默默耕耘和不懈努力，如今的博物馆扎根海上，享誉全国，名扬海外。凡是过往，皆为序章。今天，站在新时代新的历史起点，面对新的使命和挑战，我们将铭记先贤筚路蓝缕、栉风沐雨，高擎振兴中华文化之大志，打造特色，创建精品，续写辉煌篇章！

李　赣

2023 年 6 月

Preface

Located at No. 41 Chibang Road in Shanghai, the Museum of Medical History of the Chinese Medical Association, was established in July 1938 by Mr. Wang Jimin, a renowned medical historian. It became the first-ever medical history museum in China. The museum played a significant role in awakening the consciousness of patriotism in Old China (1840–1949). It emerged from the patriotic and self-strengthening endeavors of the Chinese people represented by Chinese scholars, embodying the historical, cultural, and spiritual essence of China.

The imprints of history are evident and profound, while the inheritance of culture progresses endlessly. The establishment of the museum is significant, not only in preserving and safeguarding the cultural artifacts of traditional Chinese medicine (TCM), but also in actively contributing to medical, cultural, patriotic education, and scientific popularization. Over the course of its 80-year journey, the museum has witnessed location and name changes in different stages. Throughout ups and downs, we have encountered start-up challenges, embarked on explorations, and engaged in reflective thinking, all the while experiencing the excitement of momentous progress. As we look back on the journey through the years, we see a steadfast foundation, a multitude of achievements, and an exceptionally promising future.

Eight decades of unwavering dedication have driven us on a magnificent journey. This book skillfully showcases the museum's 80-year evolution and remarkable achievements through vivid imagery and unforgettable narratives. It evokes a nostalgic yearning for the bygone era, instills admiration for our pioneers, and fills us with pride in the cultural gem that TCM represents. After generations of dedication and efforts made by museum staff, the museum has now taken root in Shanghai, earning the recognition and appreciation both at home and abroad. All that has passed is merely a prologue. Today, we are standing at the dawn of a new historical era. Confronting new missions and challenges, we should cherish the pioneering spirit of our trailblazers, who forged ahead through adversity to uphold the noble cause of revitalizing Chinese culture. With a resolute commitment to innovation and an unyielding pursuit of excellence, we shall write yet another splendid chapter in our enduring legacy!

Li Gan

June, 2023

1 上海中医药博物馆成立于 2003 年，前身是创建于 1938 年的中华医学会医史博物馆，中华医学会医史博物馆是我国最早建立的医学类主题博物馆。目前上海中医药博物馆建筑面积 6 314 m²，展览面积 4 050 m²。馆藏有中医药文物 14 000 多件，古今医籍 6 000 多册，医药期刊 3 000 多册，其中民国时期稀见中医药刊物近 400 种，基本涵盖当时全国所有发行的中医药期刊。博物馆展厅基本陈列分原始医疗活动、古代医卫遗存、历代医事管理、历代医学荟萃、养生文化撷英、近代海上中医、本草方剂鉴赏、当代岐黄新貌八个专题，反映我国 5 000 年来中医药学发展的重要史实和主要成就，在医学史教学、普及医学知识、促进中外医学交流等方面发挥重要作用。博物馆弘扬中医药文化，普及中医药科学知识，反映中医药学从形成到繁荣、从继承到创新的轨迹，是博大精深的中医药学和中医药文化的缩影。

Established in 2003, the Shanghai Museum of Traditional Chinese Medicine may trace its origins back to the Museum of Medical History of the Chinese Medical Association, which was founded in 1938. It is the first-ever medical history museum in China. Today, the museum covers a total area of 6,314 m², including exhibition halls spanning 4,050 m². It boasts an impressive collection of over 14,000 pieces of traditional Chinese medicine (TCM) relics and more than 6,000 ancient and modern medical books.

Moreover, the museum houses a vast array of over 3,000 medical journals, with nearly 400 rare TCM journals that date back to the Chinese Republican Period (1912–1949). These journals encompassed almost all the TCM journals issued nationwide during that era. The exhibition hall is divided into eight sections, each exploring different aspects of TCM's evolution and contributions.

These sections are: Primitive Medical Practice, Preserved Artifacts in Ancient Health Care, Ancient Medical Practice Management, Historical Medical Collection, Ancient Chinese Culture on Life Nurturing, Modern Chinese Medicine in Shanghai, Appreciation of Herbal Prescriptions, and New Look of Contemporary Chinese Medicine. These sections present the history and achievements of TCM development over 5,000 years, and serve a vital role in medical history teaching, the dissemination of medical knowledge, and the facilitation of medical exchanges between China and the international community.

Dedicated to promoting TCM, the museum offers a captivating showcase of the evolution, growth, legacy, and innovation within this healing practice. By delving into these diverse aspects, the museum truly epitomizes the profoundness and significance of TCM.

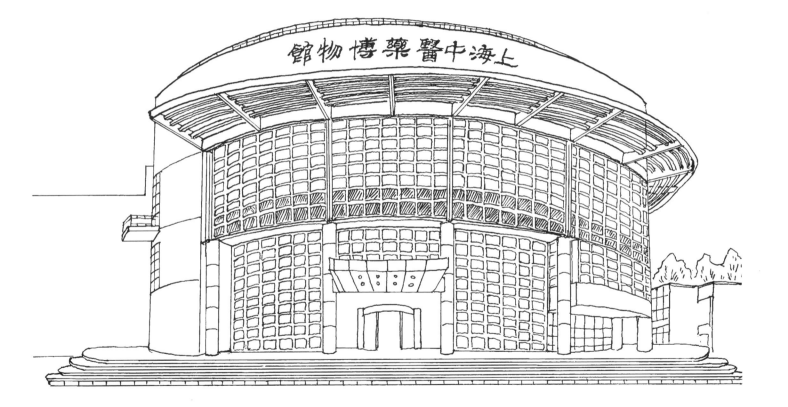

2 博物馆的创办缘由要从一本全英文的《中国医史》说起。这本《中国医史》有两位作者，王吉民和伍连德。

王吉民（1889—1972），又名嘉祥，号芸心，广东东莞人。他出生于传教士家庭，曾先后任外轮公司船医、沪杭甬铁路管理局总医官、浙江邮政管理局医官，同时在杭州开业执医。1937 年，王吉民在上海协助筹建中华医学会新会址，被选任中华医学会副会长。同年，中华医学会第四届代表大会期间，医史委员会改组为中华医史学会，王吉民任首届会长。翌年 7 月，中国第一家医学史专业博物馆——中华医学会医史博物馆在上海建成，王吉民担任馆长。抗日战争期间，医学会负责人陆续离沪，会务主要由王吉民和富文寿负责，直到抗日战争胜利。

伍连德（1879—1960），字联星，祖籍广东新宁（今台山），马来亚槟榔屿（今属马来西亚）华侨。伍连德指挥扑灭了 1910 年的东北鼠疫，之后又多次组织扑灭在东北及上海等地暴发的肺鼠疫和霍乱，为中国的卫生防疫事业做出了巨大贡献。1915 年，他与颜福庆等发起建立中华医学会，并任第二、第三届会长。在华 30 年间，伍连德先后创建 20 多所医院和医学院，培养出一批医学人才。

1935 年诺贝尔生理学或医学奖评选时，在候选人名单中，伍连德（Lien-Teh Wu）的名字赫然在列，成为首位华人诺贝尔奖候选人。

The establishment of the museum was inspired by *History of Chinese Medicine*, an English TCM literature co-authored by Wang Jimin and Lien-Teh Wu.

Wang Jimin (1889–1972), also known as Jiaxiang with the literary name (Hao) Yunxin, was born into a missionary family in Dongguan, Guangdong Province. He was firstly a doctor of a foreign steamship company and then the chief medical officer of Shanghai-Hangzhou-Ningbo Railway Administration. Later, he became a medical officer of Zhejiang Provincial Postal Administration and at the same time practiced medicine in Hangzhou. In 1937, he played a pivotal role in establishing Chinese Medical Association in a new site in Shanghai and was elected as the vice president. In the same year, during the 4th National Congress of Chinese Medical Association, the Committee of Chinese Medical History was reorganized into the Chinese Medical Association of Medical History, with Wang Jimin elected as its first president. Subsequently, in July of the following year, the Museum of Medical History of the Chinese Medical Association was established in Shanghai, marking the first specialized museum of its kind in China. Wang was also designated as the museum's president. During the Chinese People's War of Resistance Against Japanese Aggression, leaders of the association successively left Shanghai. Since then, Wang Jimin and Fu Wenshou assumed leadership of the association until China won the war.

Lien-Teh Wu (1879–1960), known by his courtesy name Lianxing, was an overseas Chinese from Penang, Malaya (now part of Malaysia), with his ancestral home traced back to Xinning (today's Taishan), Guangdong Province. In 1910, Wu took the lead to stamp out the plague outbreak in Northeastern China. Then, he also contained pneumonic plague and cholera that broke out in Northeastern China and Shanghai. Wu has greatly impacted Chinese public health and anti-epidemic initiatives.

In 1915, Wu, alongside Yan Fuqing, co-founded the Chinese Medical Association and assumed the roles of its second and third president. Throughout his three decades in China, Wu diligently established over 20 hospitals and medical schools, and nurtured a new generation of medical practitioners.

In the nomination of Nobel Prize in Physiology or Medicine in 1935, Wu's name prominently featured among the candidates, marking him as the first-ever Chinese nominee for the prestigious Nobel Prize.

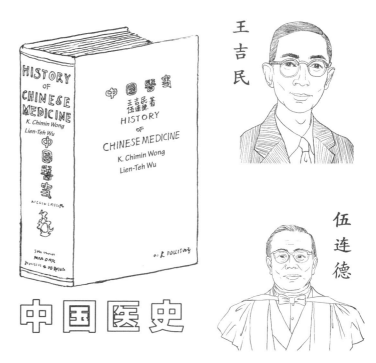

3 博物馆的建立源于王吉民与伍连德的《中国医史》，那么两人又为什么撰写此书呢？

这便要提到 1914 年美国医史学家嘉立森（Garrison）编写的《医学史》。这本书概述了世界医学的发展，全书近 700 页，其中涉及中国医学的内容却只有半页，而且存在不少错误。嘉立森评价："中国医学是完全静止的，如果我们一直到现在还受中世纪思想的指导，我们的医学可能也会和中国的一样。他们的作品很多，但是没有哪怕一丁点的科学价值……"

伍连德得知此事后，写信给该书作者质询：何以对中国医学介绍得如此微少而又做出不正确评价？

The establishment of the museum originated from the *History of Chinese Medicine* by Wang Jimin and Lien-Teh Wu. Why did they write the book? To answer this question, we have to mention another book, *An Introduction to the History of Medicine* written by the American medical historian Fielding H. Garrison in 1914. This book outlines the development of medicine in the world, with nearly 700 pages in total. However, only half a page of the book is about TCM, and there are many mistakes. "Chinese medicine is what our own medicine might be, had we been guided by medieval ideas down to the present time, that is, absolutely stationary. Its literature consists of a large number of works none of which are of the slightest scientific importance..." Garrison criticized.

After reading Garrison's book, Wu wrote him a letter, asking, "Why did you write so little about TCM? And how could you come up with those incorrect remarks on TCM?"

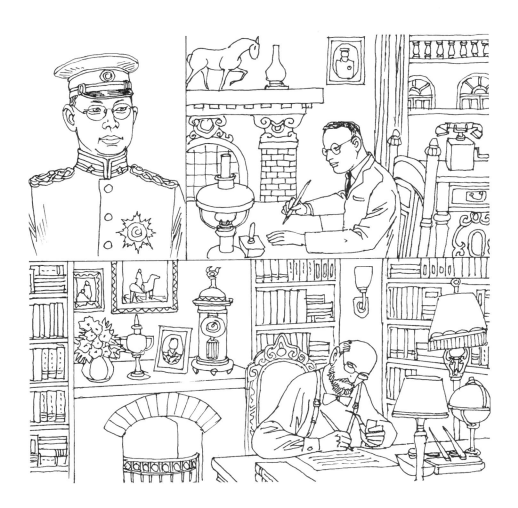

4 收到伍连德的信件后，嘉立森回信道："中医或有所长，顾未见有以西文述之者，区区半页之资料，犹属外人之作，参考无从，遂难立说，简略而误，非余之咎。"

中医既然有它的价值，为什么不向世人介绍？嘉立森的这番话激发了伍连德撰写中国医史的想法，他立刻将回信告诉了王吉民。当时王吉民才 20 多岁，担任沪杭甬铁路管理局总医官，得知此事后，便和好友伍连德联手合作，以"保存国粹，矫正外论"为初衷，用英文写成《中国医史》（*History of Chinese Medicine*）。

1929 年，嘉立森的《医学史》第 4 版中，有关中医学的内容已经增至整整 4 页，除了提到《神农本草经》《黄帝内经》和《本草纲目》等中国古典医学著作外，还增加了中医学在 20 世纪初发生的一些重大事件。文中有四次提到了伍连德的名字，还引用了伍连德 1916 年发表在《中华医学杂志》上的一篇关于控制鼠疫流行的文章。

"Traditional Chinese medicine may have its strengths, but I hardly found related materials written in English. The available content specifically addressing TCM is limited to a mere half-page, authored by a non-native individual. Without sufficient references, it becomes challenging for me to provide detailed and accurate information. Therefore, it is not my intention to make incorrect remarks about TCM in the book," expounded by Fielding H. Garrison in his correspondence to Lien-Teh Wu.

Since TCM is so valuable, why not introduce it to the rest of the world? Garrison's reply served as an impetus for Wu to undertake the compilation of a book about the history of TCM. He promptly relayed Garrison's comments to Wang Jimin, who then was in his 20s and served as the chief medical officer of Shanghai-Hangzhou-Ningbo Railway Administration. Upon learning the letter, Wang decided to work together with Wu to write the book, *History of Chinese Medicine*, in English. Their aim was to "conserve Chinese quintessence and rectify foreign bias".

In 1929, the 4th edition of *An Introduction to the History of Medicine* by Garrison was published. It featured a notable augmentation in the coverage of TCM, encompassing a comprehensive span of four pages. In addition to a series of Chinese medical classics, such as *Shennong's Classic of Materia Medica* (*Shen Nong Ben Cao Jing*), *Huangdi's Internal Classic* (*Huang Di Nei Jing*) and *Compendium of Materia Medica* (*Ben Cao Gang Mu*), the book also introduces some major events that happened in the

Chinese medical sector in the early 20th century. In his book, Garrison aptly mentioned Wu's name on four distinct occasions. He even cited a paper published by Wu in 1916 in the *Traditional Medical Journal of China* about controlling plague.

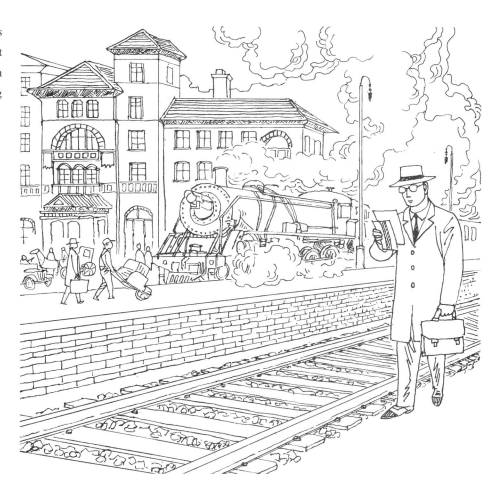

5《中国医史》全书分为上篇和下篇，上篇约占 1/4，由王吉民撰写；下篇约占 3/4，由伍连德起草。

上篇分四个时期重点介绍了中医的进化和发展，分别为古代或传说时期（Ancient or Legendary Period，公元前 2697—前 1122 年）、有历史记载的或黄金时期（Historical or Golden Period，公元前 1121—960 年）、中世纪或争鸣时期（Medieval or Controversial Period，961—1800 年）、现代或转折时期（Modern or Transitional Period，1801—1936 年）。下篇则重点介绍了西医传入中国的进程，自 1800 年起，西医与中国的早期接触、教会行医、设立医院、推广医学教育、治理黑死病、海港检疫等。文中引用了诸多第一手史料，对西医在我国逐步成长的历史做了较为翔实的记载，留下了不可或缺的重要医史资料。

该书向世界介绍了中国传统医学的历史成就，维护了中医的地位和尊严，同时也提出中医与西医是研究同一目标的两个不同学术体系，既要保持传统，又要科学现代化发展。

The *History of Chinese Medicine* is divided into two parts: Part One, written by Wang Jimin, occupies approximately 1/4 of the book; Part Two, drafted by Lien-Teh Wu, accounts for the remaining 3/4.

Part One focuses on the evolution of TCM across four distinct periods: the Ancient or Legendary Period (2697 BCE–1121 BCE), the Historical or Golden Period (1121 BCE–960), the Medieval or Controversial Period (961–1800), and the Modern or Transitional Period (1801–1936). Part Two, on the other hand, highlights the introduction of Western medicine to China since the 19th century. It encompasses various aspects, such as the early interactions between Western and Chinese medicine, the church's medical practices, the establishment of hospitals, the promotion of medical education, as well as the treatment of the Black Death and port quarantine, etc. The book cites numerous first-hand historical materials and provides a comprehensive and unbiased account of Western medicine's development in China, preserving vital and irreplaceable records for the history of medicine. The book not only presents TCM's historical accomplishments to the world, but also upholds the esteemed status and dignity of TCM. Furthermore, it advocates that Western medicine and TCM are two distinct academic systems, yet sharing a common focus on studying the human body. It emphasizes the importance of preserving their respective traditions while embracing scientific modernization.

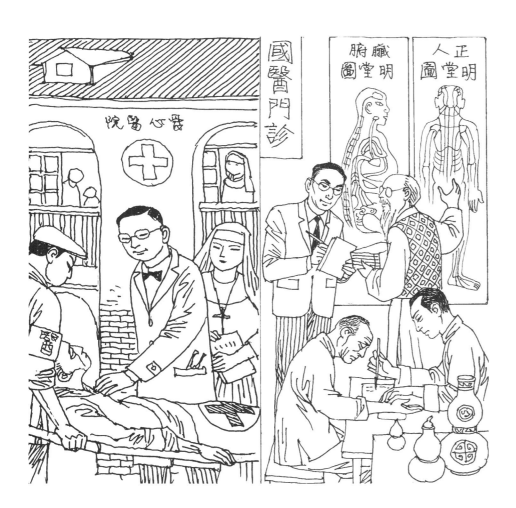

院醫心慈

國醫門診

腑臟圖堂明

人正圖堂明

6 王吉民和伍连德写成《中国医史》非常不容易，遇到重重困难。撰写期间，他们四处奔走，广泛搜集历代医史资料，查阅典籍，潜心整理研究。

伍连德在《中国医史》第一版序言中说："我们只能找到极为稀少的信息碎片。我们不得不查阅和梳理广泛散布在几个国家用多种语言写成的无数杂志、书籍、报告等，并对所需信息进行仔细审查。"

从 1915 年王吉民和伍连德萌生写书的初心开始，耗时多年，直到 1932 年才编写成书。

Wang Jimin and Lien-Teh Wu faced great hardship in compiling the *History of Chinese Medicine.* They endeavored to amass an extensive array of materials for Chinese medical history. They also consulted Chinese medical classics, collating and studying the collections with their whole hearts.

Eventually, the inaugural edition of *History of Chinese Medicine* was published. Wu stated in the preface: "In the first place, scant and disjointed sources of information alone were available. Innumerable journals, books, reports, etc. in many languages and widely scattered over several countries had to be consulted and combed, and the required information carefully checked."

Since Wang and Wu were sparked by the idea of writing the book in 1915, it took several years of hard work until the book was finally completed in 1932.

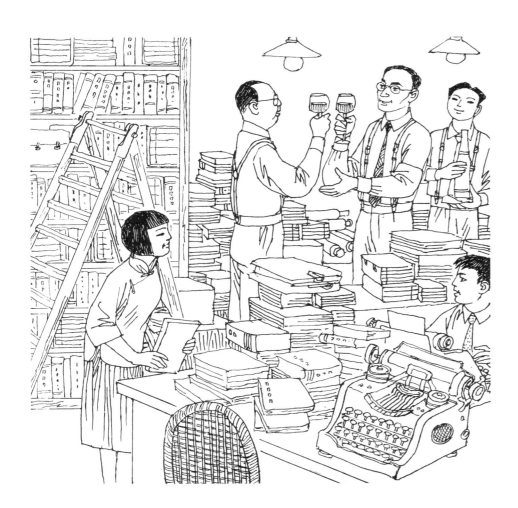

7 经过两位先生的不懈努力，《中国医史》终于在 1932 年由天津印字馆出版。后经过修订完善，1936 年由上海全国海港检疫管理处再版。2009 年，根据王吉民之女王慕兰女士提供的 1936 年版本为底本，由上海辞书出版社重新影印出版，韩启德院士在这一版《中国医史》的序言中说道："回溯医学史，就是对医学价值的精神回归。"

《中国医史》的出版，不仅填补了中国医学对外交流的空白，而且更让世界对中医药有了基本和系统的认识，在世界医学史上留下浓墨重彩的一笔，迄今仍被许多国外知名图书馆收藏。英国科技史学家李约瑟博士在《美国中医》杂志上发表文章赞扬此书"几乎是西方医学史家所知道的唯一的书"。

《中国医史》一书影响深远，2000 年由卫生部组织修撰，人民卫生出版社出版的《中国医学通史》，其中原始资料大多源于王伍二人的《中国医史》原书。

As a result of the unremitting efforts of Wang Jimin and Lien-Teh Wu, in 1932, the inaugural edition of *History of Chinese Medicine* was finally published by the Tianjin Printing House. Following subsequent revisions and enhancements, in 1936 the second edition of the book was reprinted by National Quarantine Service in Shanghai. In 2009, *History of Chinese Medicine* was photocopied and reprinted by Shanghai Lexicographical Publishing House based on the 1936 edition provided by Wang Mulan, daughter of Wang Jimin. "The retrospective study of medical history represents a spiritual return to the core values of the medical field.", Han Qide, academician of Chinese Academy of Sciences, wrote in the preface.

This masterpiece, the *History of Chinese Medicine*, holds a significant position in world medical history and is collected by famous libraries worldwide. Beyond bridging the communication gap between Chinese medical history and world medical history, the book also serves to make people all over the world understand the basics of TCM in a systematic way. Dr. Joseph Needham, a British expert on the history of science and technology, lauded this book as "practically the only known book to Western medical historians" in an article published in the *American Journal of Chinese Medicine*.

The influence of the book on Chinese medical history is far-reaching. *A General History of Chinese Medicine*, compiled by Ministry of Health of the People's Republic of China (now National Health Commission of the People's Republic of China) and published by People's Medical Publishing House in 2000, heavily drew upon this book as a primary source of reference material.

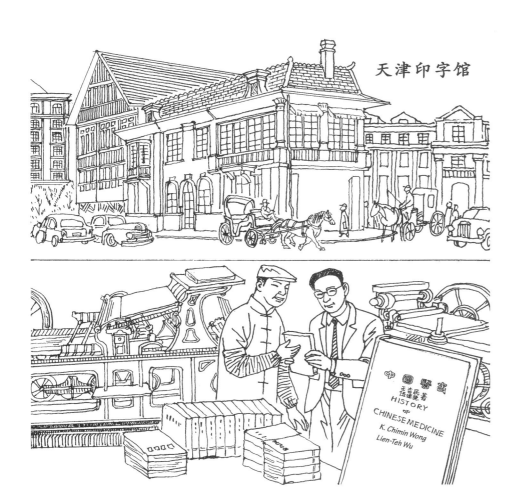

天津印字馆

中國醫書
王吉民 著
伍連德
HISTORY
OF
CHINESE MEDICINE
K. Chimin Wong
Lien-Teh Wu

8 《中国医史》成书的过程，让王吉民意识到研究医学史的重要性，尤其是通过研究中国医学史，发扬中国传统医学。

1937 年 4 月，中华医学会第四届代表大会在上海召开。大会有建议将各分会升为独立学会，于是医史委员会重新改组为中华医史学会，同时仍为中华医学会的医史分组，王吉民被推选为会长。1940 年 12 月，中华医学会加入国际医史学会，成为会员之一，并于执行委员会中列席。

中华医史学会成立初期通过了 6 条建议：① 搜集有关医史材料。② 发行医史杂志。③ 翻译中医典籍。④ 刊行会员医史著作。⑤ 建立中医图书馆。⑥ 筹设医史博物馆。其中所提及的医史博物馆便是后来的上海中医药博物馆。

在这次大会期间，王吉民组织举办了医史文献展览会，由中华医学会拨款 300 元，作为购置大会时医史展览物品的经费。此次医史文献展览会被看作是中华医史学会成立 5 年间最值得纪念的事迹。

While writing *History of Chinese Medicine*, Wang Jimin recognized the significance of studying medical history, especially Chinese medical history. In doing so, TCM could be carried forward.

In April 1937, the 4th National Congress of the Chinese Medical Association was held in Shanghai, where a proposal was put forth to promote the Association's branches into independent associations. Building upon this proposal, the Committee of Chinese Medical History, a branch of the Chinese Medical Association at the time, was reorganized and became the Chinese Medical Association of Medical History. Wang Jimin was elected as the president of this newly formed association. In December 1940, the Chinese Medical Association joined the International Society for the History of Medicine, becoming one of its members and serving on its executive committee.

During the early stage of the Chinese Medical Association of Medical History, six proposals were approved, including the collection of materials for medical history, the publication of medical history magazines, the translation of TCM classics, the publication of works by association members, the establishment of a TCM library, and preparations to set up a medical history museum. This museum mentioned above was later known as the Shanghai Museum of Traditional Chinese Medicine.

During this congress, Wang Jimin organized the Exhibition of Medical History Documents, utilizing 300 silver dollars allocated by the Chinese

Medical Association for the acquisition of exhibits. This exhibition was hailed as the most significant event in the five years since the establishment of the association.

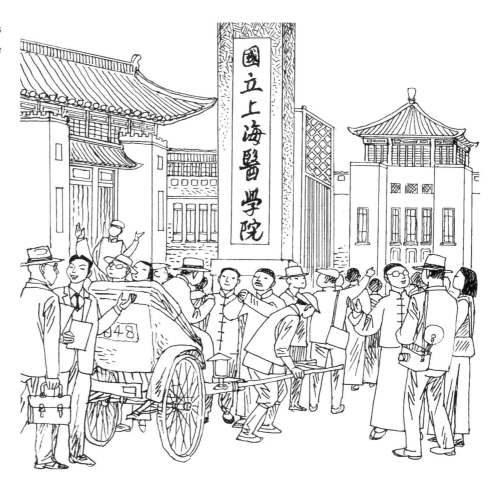

9 医史文献展览会在枫林桥的国立上海医学院松德堂内举办，经过多位中医人、各地收藏家 30 余人共同合作，搜罗全国及各国的宝贵文献，所陈列的物品达千余种，主要分为四类。① 图书类：史传、目录、译著、期刊、珍籍。② 画像类：名医肖像、医事图书、表册。③ 物品类：外科仪器、针灸器具、内科用具、药用器皿、雕刻塑像。④ 医俗类：医药神像、神马、仙方、符咒及其他。

展览会上珍品众多，其中有德、法、英、美、日等国学者研究中医中药的巨著数十种，并且都增加了中文提要说明，如 1735 年法译《脉决》及各国译本的《本草纲目》，1882 年创刊的中文《西医新报》，1905 年出版的中医最早的杂志《医学报》；名画如故宫博物院藏的宋李唐《灸艾图》，天津达仁堂主人所藏的医药祖师图，平时不轻易示人的物品，均在此次展览会上陈列。

The Exhibition of Medical History Documents took place in the esteemed Songde Hall of Shanghai Medical College at Fenglin Bridge, thanks to the collaborative efforts of over 30 renowned TCM scholars and collectors in China. Notably, the event saw the active participation of numerous TCM practitioners, who contributed valuable documents from both China and the rest of the world. The exhibition showcased an impressive array of over a thousand exhibits, which can be categorized as follows: ① Books: historical biographies, catalogs, translations, periodicals and treasured classics. ② Images: portraits featuring esteemed doctors, medical books and lists. ③ Tools and artifacts: surgical instruments, acupuncture and moxibustion tools, internal medicine tools, medicinal utensils, and sculptures. ④ Items of medical customs: statues of famous doctors, divine horses, prescriptions with great efficacy, and spells, etc.

The exhibition housed numerous precious collections, including dozens of TCM masterpieces authored by scholars from Germany, France, the United Kingdom, the United States and Japan. All collections were accompanied by Chinese annotations. Among the remarkable exhibits were books and journals such as the French translation of *Pulse Diagnosis* (*Mai Jue*) in 1735, various language versions of *Compendium of Materia Medica*, the *Medical News* published in 1882, the *Medical Journal* published in 1905, as well as celebrated paintings like *The Moxibustion* by Li Tang of the Song Dynasty, which is housed in the Palace Museum, and *The Portrait of the Forefather of Medicine*, collected by the owner of Tianjin Darentang Pharmaceutical Factory.

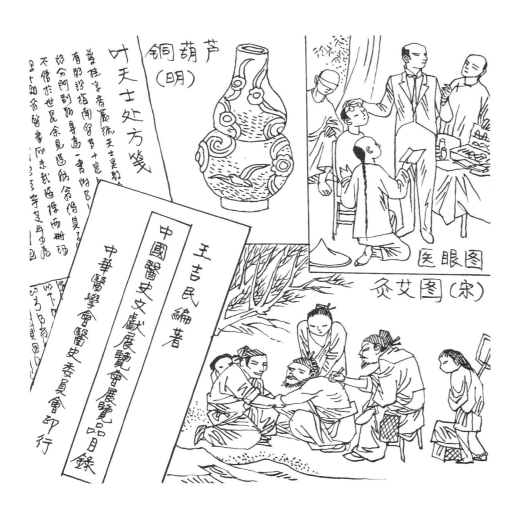

10 1937 年 4 月 7 日，《申报》刊登了医史文献展览会的报道，并公布展览会将在 4 月 7 日下午 2 点至 4 点及 4 月 8 日上午 9 点至 12 点，向公众开放，邀请社会人士参观。

得知此消息之后，社会各界前往参观的人络绎不绝，中医界人士尤为踊跃，到会参观者有三四千人之多。

On April 7, 1937, the *Shen Bao Newspaper* published a report about the Exhibition of Medical History Documents, stating that the exhibition would be open to the public from 2 p.m. to 4 p.m. on April 7, and 9 a.m. to 12 a.m. on April 8.

Upon hearing this announcement, approximately three or four thousand visitors from various sectors of society, particularly the TCM community, eagerly flocked to the exhibition.

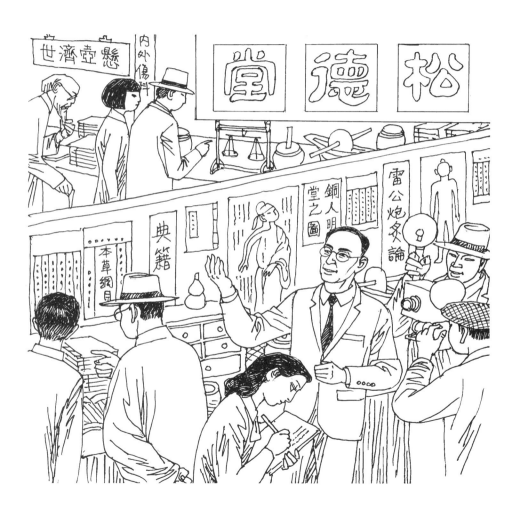

11 除了举办医史文献展览会外，王吉民还在中华医史学会第四届第一次全体会议上，做了题为《组织中华医史博物馆之建议》的演讲。他明确了博物馆保存、研究、教育的三大职能，并提出以此次医史文献展览会所搜集的展品为起点，往后每年由医史学会指定的款项，随时收购。他坚信五年十载之后，此馆成绩一定相当可观。

中华医史博物馆选址上海，也是经过了王吉民的一番考量。他认为中华医学会的会员多达三千人，各地分会有数十余，遍布全国各个省市，非常便于搜集资料。而上海，交通便利，职员也多，便于管理，参观及研究都很方便。

中华医学会医史博物馆便由此孕育而生。

In addition to holding the Exhibition of Medical History Documents, Wang Jimin also gave a speech titled "Suggestions on Organizing a Museum for the Chinese Medical History of the Chinese Medical Association" at the First Plenary Meeting of the 4th Session of the Chinese Medical Association. Wang defined the three functions of the museum as preservation, research and education. He further proposed that the museum utilize the current exhibition's artifacts as a foundational collection and continue to expand its holdings through annual allocations from the association. He firmly believed that, the collection of the museum would be extensive and impressive a few years later.

The new site of the museum in Shanghai was also the result of Wang's consideration and effort. Given that the Chinese Medical Association had as many as 3,000 members and dozens of branches spanning the entire nation, an environment conducive to the gathering of medical literature was fostered. Additionally, the Shanghai Branch had a sizable staff and benefited from convenient transportation, which facilitated smoother management, visits and research endeavors.

Hence, the Museum of Medical History of the Chinese Medical Association was formally established in Shanghai.

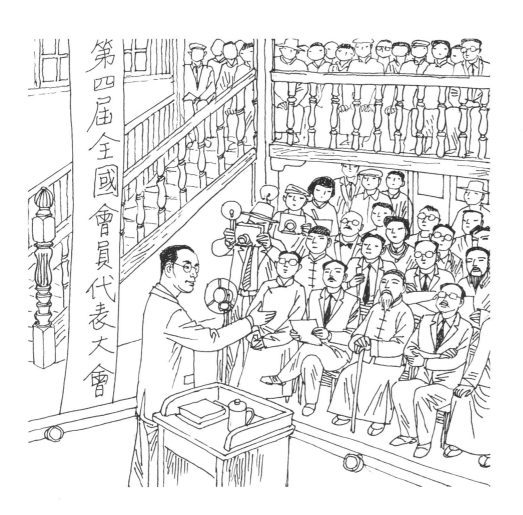

12 1937 年 4 月，医史文献展览会闭幕，归还了部分借展物品后，剩余的物品便成了博物馆藏品的核心，随后博物馆又得到各方的捐赠、借用以及零星添购。1938 年 7 月，中国第一家医史博物馆正式对外开放。博物馆刚成立的时候有陈列品约 400 件，包括医事图画、手笔、明堂图表、书法、印章、名医肖像、仙方、药神、各种药瓶、铜器、象牙雕刻、医药用具、外科器械，以及其他艺术物品等。

Following this exhibition in April 1937, part of the borrowed exhibits was returned, with the remaining exhibits being the core of this museum's collection. Later, in addition to receiving exhibits from various sources, staff in the museum also borrowed and purchased exhibits.

The first museum of medical history in China officially opened to the public in July 1938! When the museum was first established, there were about 400 exhibits, including medical drawings, writings, meridians and acupoints charts, calligraphy works, seals, portraits of famous doctors, prescriptions with great efficacy, statues of famous doctors, medicine bottles, cooper ware, ivory carvings, medical instruments, surgical instruments and various other artworks.

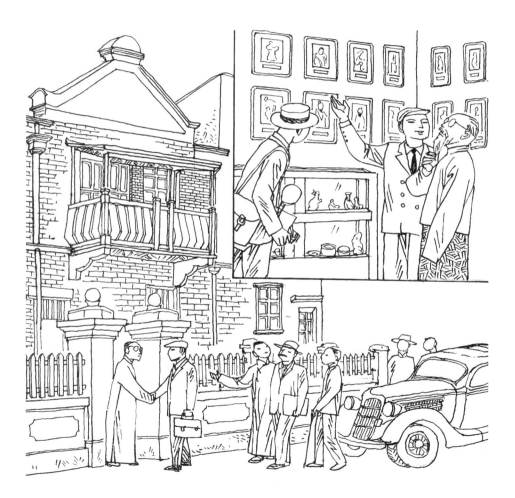

13 1937 年"八一三"事变后，上海处于日本侵略军战火的严重威胁之中，环境恶劣。1941 年太平洋战争爆发，日军进驻租界，上海被日本人控制，中华医学会这样的文化机构自然也成为侵略者的垂涎对象。在日军侵占上海期间，王吉民考虑到所收藏的中医学珍本与文物的安全，将它们分别转移，保存于留沪国际友人、同道、教友家中。至日本投降，这些珍贵之物均得以完好无损地保护下来。

Following the August 13th Incident in 1937, Shanghai faced a grave threat from the Japanese aggressors. With the outbreak of the Pacific War in 1941, Japanese troops took control of Shanghai and occupied the concessions. Amidst this occupation, the Japanese invaders cast their greedy eyes on cultural institutions such as the Chinese Medical Association. In response, Wang Jimin took action to safeguard the valuable books and cultural relics of TCM. He arranged for their transfer to the homes of trusted foreign friends, fellows, and co-religionists in Shanghai. Due to his efforts, the precious collections remained intact and preserved until Japan's surrender.

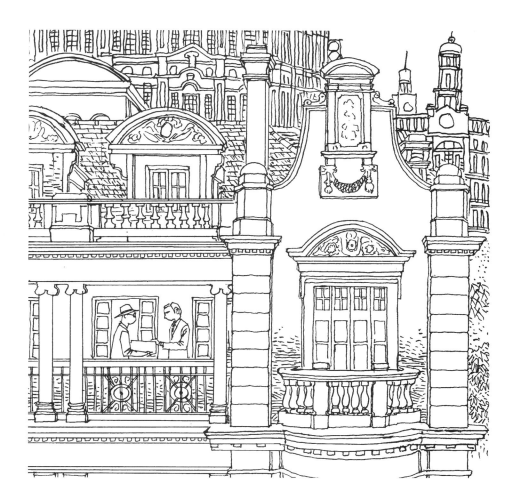

14 杭州智果寺住持清华禅师精研岐黄，一生藏书颇丰，曾编印《清华医室珍藏医书类目》，收录医书千余种，分 12 类，每类摘取一二种，提要钩元。1936 年，禅师涅槃，遗嘱将所藏医书捐赠给图书馆，但他的裔僧欲将藏书出售，消息传出，各路书商纷纷争购。王吉民四处托人去智果寺商谈，几经周折，最终决议有价转让给中华医史学会。王吉民用伍连德捐款中的一部分购得这批藏书，有 400 余种，其中不乏孤本、珍本。

智果寺旧址位于杭州市西湖区葛岭路 1 号，现仅存寺门及几级石阶，被列为杭州市文物保护点。

Zen Master Qinghua, abbot of the Zhiguo Temple in Hangzhou, devoted his entire life to studying TCM. He amassed a vast collection of books with life-long efforts and complied the *Catalog of Medical Books in the Collection of Qinghua Physician's Office* (*Qing Hua Yi Shi Zhen Cang Yi Shu Lei Mu*), which records more than a thousand types of medical books that are divided into 12 categories. Qinghua carefully selected one or two representative medical books from each category, exploring the essence and explaining the gist. In 1936, Master Qinghua passed away. He left his will to donate all his collections to a library, but his successor intended to sell them all instead. Once the news broke, booksellers eagerly scrambled to purchase the books. Wang Jimin sought the assistance of middlemen to negotiate with the Zhiguo Temple. After twists and turns, he won the deal with the temple on compensable transfer of the collections to the Chinese Medical Association of Medical History. With a part of the donation from Lien-Teh Wu, Wang acquired approximately 400 types of books, including rare and unique copies.

Zhiguo Temple's former location was at No.1 Geling Road, Xihu District, Hangzhou. Presently, only the temple gate and a few stone steps remain at the site, which has been designated as a protected cultural relic in Hangzhou.

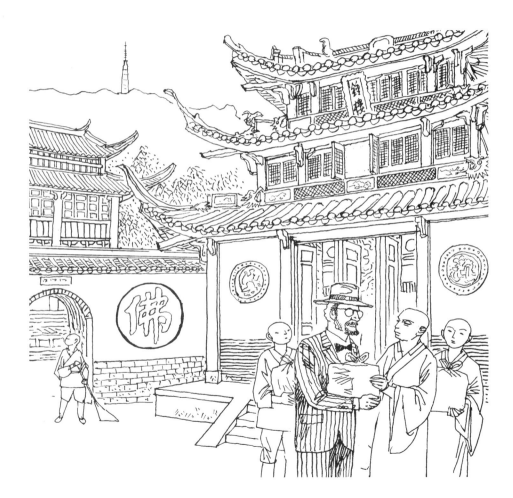

15 1942 年，王吉民冒着生命危险亲自赴杭，设法搬运清华藏书。到了杭州，鉴于当时日本人对外国人还有三分顾忌，于是他托之江大学（1952 年全国高校调整院系，之江大学各个院系分别并入同济大学、上海财经学院、浙江大学等高校）外籍教授马先生去搬运图书。马教授每日自秦望山入城，乘坐汽车，穿行于日本侵略者明晃晃的刺刀下，一车一车搬运，如此费时 1 个月，才将藏书暂存至之江大学。再以学校名义打包交转运公司寄到中华医学会，前后花费约 3 个月时间。

In 1942, Wang Jimin risked his life to go to Hangzhou for transferring Qinghua's collections. Recognizing the comparatively more tolerant behavior of the Japanese military towards foreigners, Wang entrusted Professor Ma to transport the collections upon his arrival. Ma was a foreign professor of Hangchow University, whose divisions later were merged into several universities, including Tongji University, Shanghai University of Finance and Economics, and Zhejiang University, in accordance with the adjustment of national college system in 1952.

Every day, Professor Ma drove to the city from Qinwang Mountain. He braved the presence of armed Japanese aggressors with menacing bayonets while transferring the books repeatedly. After a month of unwavering efforts, he successfully retrieved and temporarily stored all the collections in Hangchow University. Subsequently, he packed up the books and arranged for an express company to ship them to the Chinese Medical Association under the name of Hangchow University. The entire process spanned approximately 3 months.

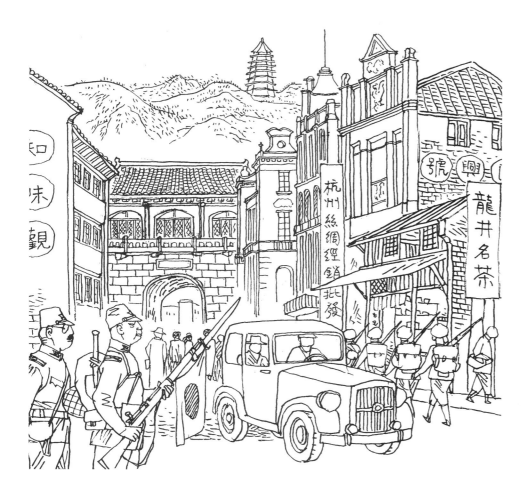

16 1943 年，王吉民与丁济民谈论起中国医史文物的相关问题，提及多年前北平（现为北京）某古董铺有一具针灸铜人，应是满族某旗家传数代的珍品。可惜当时囊中羞涩，没有足够资金为博物馆买下它。王吉民一直对此深感遗憾。丁济民（1912—1979）是江苏武进人，为江南医界宗师丁甘仁之嫡孙，家学渊源。他得知此事后，同样引以为憾，因为上海公私收藏家虽多，但未必有收藏针灸铜人的，便表示只要古董铺没有将铜人卖出去，他愿想办法出资购置。

In 1943, when Wang Jimin talked to Ding Jimin about relics of Chinese medical history, he mentioned an acupuncture copper figure that he had come across in an antique shop in Beijing several years ago. He suggested that it should be a family heirloom belonging to one of the Eight Banners of Manchu. Unfortunately, he deeply regretted not being able to purchase it due to his tight budget. Ding Jimin (1912–1979) was born in Wujin, Jiangsu Province. He grew up in a family closely bonded to TCM, as he was the legitimate grandson of Ding Ganren, a renowned TCM master in Jiangnan, the regions south of the Yangtze River. He also felt sorry upon hearing the story. Although there were many public and private collectors in Shanghai, it was uncertain whether they would be willing to acquire an acupuncture copper figure. Therefore, Ding expressed his willingness to purchase the copper figure as long as the antique shop had not sold it out.

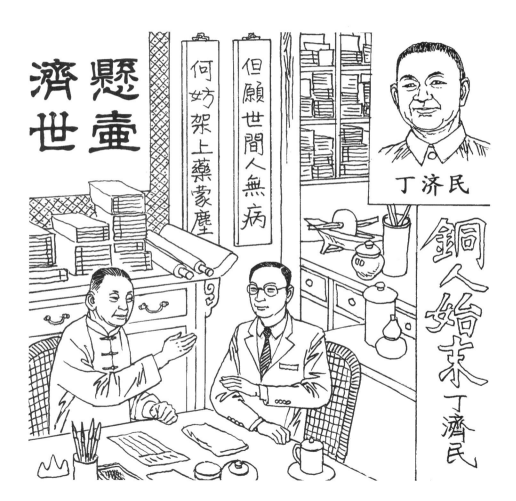

丁济民

懸壺濟世

何妨架上藥蒙塵

但願世間人無病

銅人始末 丁濟民

17 1944年，王吉民写信托北平李友松医师去古董铺访购，幸而原物犹存，但因物主离开北平和售价高涨的关系，几经周折才将它买下。正值战乱，交通运输极为不便，铜人被买下后便只能暂时搁置北平。一直等到王吉民的友人王顺和先生冒着危险趁来沪之便，设法将铜人一道带来上海。

In 1944, Wang Jimin wrote to Li Yousong, a physician from Beijing, requesting his assistance in acquiring the copper figure from the antique shop. Fortunately, the copper figure remained unsold, but purchasing it proved to be a challenging endeavor for Li: the owner had already left Beijing and the price of the copper figure was skyrocketing. Furthermore, due to the transportation difficulties caused by the ongoing war, the copper figure had to be temporarily stored in Beijing until Wang Shunhe, a friend of Wang Jimin, courageously undertook the risk of bring it to Shanghai, where Wang Jimin resided.

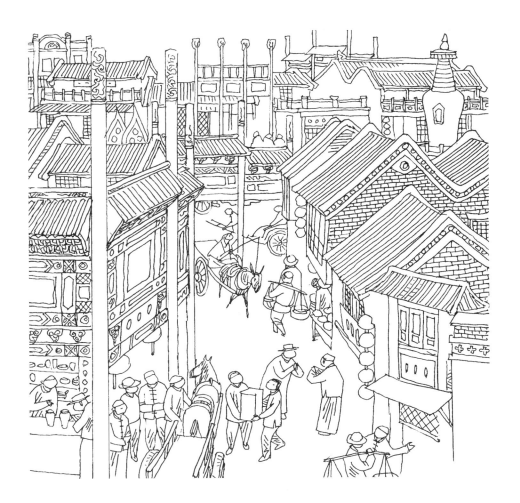

18 因战乱时期，交通格外困难，从北平到上海，一路过关涉卡，多次遇险，因种种不便，运输铜人产生的意外费用几乎超过购价，这部分支出同样由丁济民承担。事后，丁济民感慨道："这一躯并不高大的铜人，在承平时候，由平运沪，真是轻而易举之事。而在今日，觉得比搬一座大山还难。"

Transportation was highly inconvenient during the war, with countless checkpoints and risks along the route from Beijing to Shanghai. Ding Jimin had to bear the unexpected transportation cost, which nearly exceeded the price of the copper figure itself. "In times of peace, it was a simple task to transport the copper figure of medium height from Beijing to Shanghai. But now, it was like challenging as moving a mountain." exclaimed Ding Jimin afterwards.

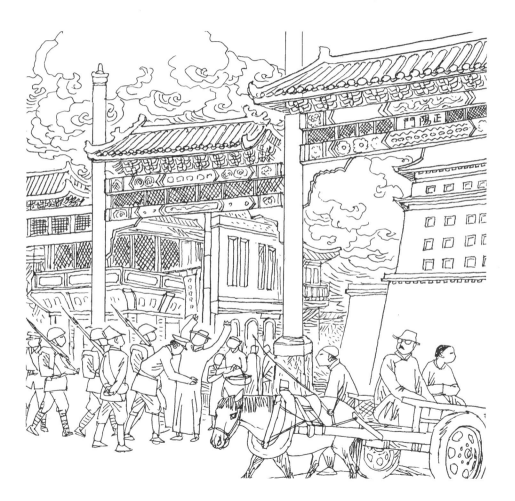

19 清乾隆针灸铜人入藏中华医学会医史博物馆，这是最好的归宿，正如丁济民先生在中华医史学会演讲"铜人始末"时所言："始于医官院，终于博物馆。"铜人的展出，使更多大众对针灸学发展有所了解，知晓《医宗金鉴》的编写过程以及铜人背后的故事。如今，这具清乾隆针灸铜人已成为上海中医药博物馆的镇馆之宝。

The Museum of Medical History of the Chinese Medical Association is now home of the acupuncture copper figure that dates back to the Qianlong Period of the Qing Dynasty. In his speech titled "The Whole Story of the Copper Figure" to the Chinese Medical Association of Medical History, Ding Jimin revealed that the copper figure was initially introduced at the Imperial Academy of Medicine before being permanently housed in the museum. The exhibition of this copper figure has provided valuable insights into the evolution of acupuncture and moxibustion, the compilation of *Golden Mirror of Medicine* (*Yi Zong Jin Jian*), and the intriguing history of the figure. Today, the copper figure stands as the most prized possession of the Shanghai Museum of Traditional Chinese Medicine.

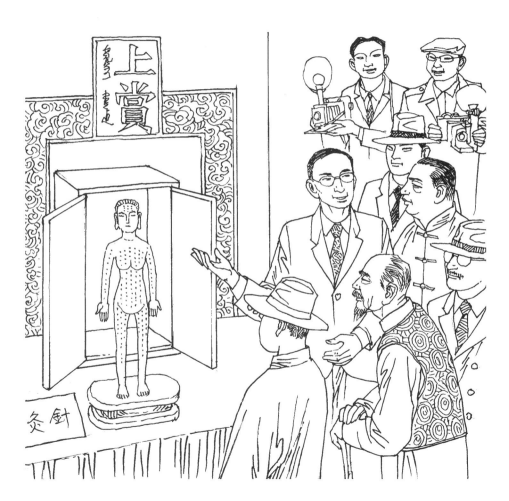

20 既然是镇馆之宝，那它有什么独特之处呢？早在清乾隆初年，太医院吴谦等人奉旨纂修《医宗金鉴》，全书共 90 卷，分为 15 个部分，采集了自春秋战国至明清历代医著精华，为一部大型综合性医书。参与修书的都是经过认真挑选而录用的精通医学、兼通文理的人员。书成之后，乾隆皇帝下令嘉奖参与编书人员，每人晋升一级，并赐针灸铜人和所修《医宗金鉴》一部。乾隆十四年（1749 年）太医院将此巨著列为医学生的教科书。入藏博物馆的铜人原为《医宗金鉴》誊录官福海之物，誊录官主要负责誊写、抄录稿件。这具铜人装于一锦盒中，黄铜质，暗铜色，高 45.8 cm，宽 22.8 cm，厚 16 cm，为一直立裸体老妇人形象。体表刻有腧穴而无腧穴名，内空而不可开合，更无脏腑诸事。

As the most prized possession of the museum, what's so unique about it? In the early years of Qianlong Period, the Qing Dynasty, by order of the emperor, Wu Qian and his colleagues from the Imperial Academy of Medicine compiled the *Golden Mirror of Medicine*. This remarkable work consists of 90 volumes divided into 15 parts. It is a large-scale comprehensive medical book, collecting the essence of medical works from the Spring and Autumn Period and Warring States Period to the Ming and Qing Dynasties.

The professionals chosen for the compilation underwent rigorous selection, demonstrating expertise not only in medicine but also in liberal arts and sciences. After the book was completed, Emperor Qianlong ordered to commend the personnel involved in compiling the book. Each was promoted and given an acupuncture copper figure and a copy of *Golden Mirror of Medicine*.

In the 14th year of Qianlong (1749), this masterpiece was listed as a textbook for medical students. The acupuncture copper figure collected in the museum was originally owned by Fuhai, an imperial transcriber, who was mainly responsible for documenting materials and copying manuscripts. This acupuncture copper figure with a dark copper color is elegantly encased in brocade, portraying an elderly naked woman standing upright. Measuring 45.8 cm in height, 22.8 cm in width, and 16 cm in thickness, the figure is adorned with intricately engraved acupuncture points, albeit without their corresponding names. It is not meant to be opened, as it is hollow inside and devoid of any zang-fu organs.

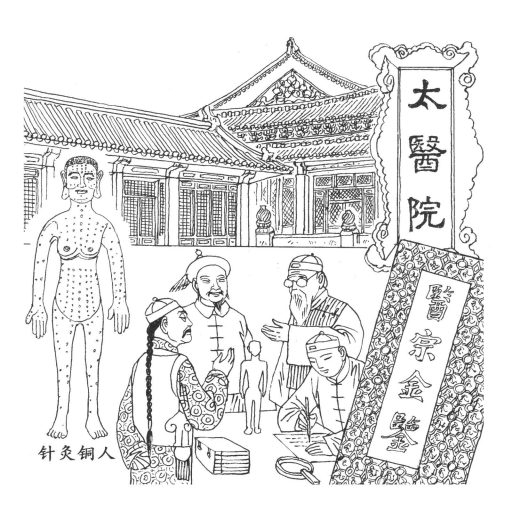

针灸铜人

太醫院

醫宗金鑒

21 清乾隆针灸铜人入藏博物馆后，引来世人关注。原来，早在北宋王惟一应诏编写《新铸铜人腧穴针灸图经》后，还主持制造了历史上最早的针灸铜人，名为天圣铜人，一座置于东京（今河南开封）相国寺仁济殿内，另一座置于医官院。铜人以成年男子为形象，与真人同等大小，内藏脏器，外壳可拆，体表刻有穴位与名称，穴位深约 1.2 分。铜人可作针灸教学之用，考试时将铜人体表封腊，体内注水或水银，取穴准确则针入水出，反之则无法刺入。这两具铜人直接用于医学知识的传授和演示，在我国古代针灸教育中发挥了重要作用，这是针灸史上的创举。靖康年间，金兵攻陷东京，一座铜人流落襄阳；另一座被金兵掳掠到北方后下落不明。

The collection of acupuncture copper figure attracted wide attention. In fact, as early as the Northern Song Dynasty, Wang Weiyi wrote *Illustrated Manual of Acupuncture Points on the Bronze Figure (Xin Zhu Tong Ren Shu Xue Zhen Jiu Tu Jing)* at the behest of the emperor, and he also presided over the production of the earliest acupuncture copper figures called Tiansheng. Two Tiansheng acupuncture copper figures were produced-one resided in the Renji Hall of Xiangguo Temple in Dongjing (now Kaifeng, Henan Province), and the other found its place in the Imperial Academy of Medicine. These figures resemble adult men in image and size. They were constructed with the capability to be opened, revealing zang-fu organs within. On the surface, there're acupuncture points with names engraved at a depth of 0.4 cm. They served as teaching aids for acupuncture lessons. For use in exams, water or mercury was introduced into the figures and the surfaces were sealed with wax. During exams, if the acupuncture points were selected accurately, the needles would enter and the water or mercury would be forced out, otherwise the needles would not penetrate. These two acupuncture copper figures were directly used for medical demonstrations and played an important role in acupuncture education in ancient China. They are a remarkable innovation in the history of acupuncture. However, during the Jingkang Period (1126–1127), troops from the Jin Dynasty captured Dongjing, leading to the relocation of the acupuncture copper figure to Xiangyang; the other one was plundered and taken to the north, and its whereabouts remain unknown.

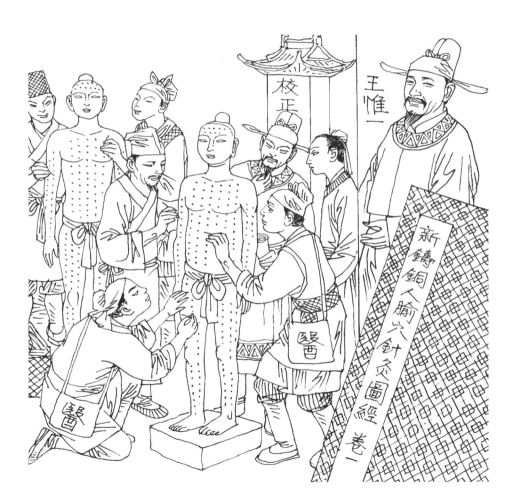

校正

王惟一

新鑄銅人腧穴針灸圖經卷一

22 抗日战争时期，在王吉民和同仁们的努力下，克服战乱等困难，博物馆的藏品非但没有损失，反而日渐丰富。1946年12月12日，中华医史学会在中华医学会大礼堂举行庆祝抗日战争胜利博物馆展览，一则庆祝抗战胜利，河山光复；二则向西方同道介绍中国医药文化，陈列展品均十分珍贵。据记录，到会者约80人，其中30余人为盟军驻沪医务人员，济济一堂，实为盛事。因这次展览会为招待盟邦英美军医的军官而设，故未公开。《医史杂志》1947年第1期登载了此次特别展览会的合影。

Thanks to the efforts of Wang Jimin and his colleagues, the museum's collections were safeguarded from devastating losses and even became increasingly abundant during the Chinese People's War of Resistance Against Japanese Aggression. On December 12, 1946, the Chinese Medical Association of Medical History organized an exhibition in its auditorium, celebrating China's victory in the war and its liberation, while also promoting TCM culture to Western medical peers. The exhibited items were of immense value. According to records, this remarkable exhibition attracted around 80 visitors, with over 30 being medical officers from the Anti-fascist Alliance stationed in Shanghai. As the event was exclusively for entertaining British and American military medical officers, it was not open to the public. Nonetheless, photos of this special exhibition were published in the *Journal of Medical History*, Issue No.1 of 1947.

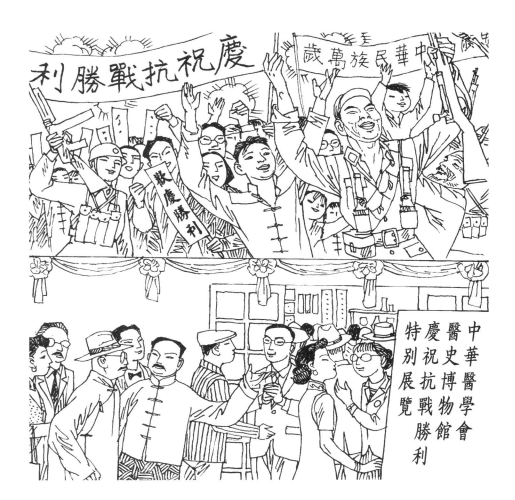

23 1947 年 12 月 20～21 日，中华医史学会与中华医学会联合举办中国医史文物展览会，展品之多，规模之大，皆远胜于前。参加此次展览会的来宾众多，包括私人医史收藏家、大学教授、艺术家、考古学家、历史学家、医校学生及中西名医等。展览品大体可以分为博物、书籍、书画三大类，博物方面，有石器、铜器、瓷器、漆器、象牙、雕刻、竹刻、木刻、丝织品及泥塑等；书籍方面，有宋元明清以来孤本珍籍；书画方面，有宋元明清以来名医、名人珍贵作品。

The Exhibition of Chinese Medical History Relics was jointly organized by the Chinese Medical Association of Medical History and Chinese Medical Association from December 20 to December 21, 1947. Distinguished by its extensive collection and significant scale, this exhibition surpassed its predecessors, attracting numerous guests, including private collectors of medical history, professors of universities, artists, archeologists, historians, students of medical schools, and famous doctors of Chinese and Western medicine. Exhibits could be generally divided into three categories: books, calligraphy works, paintings, and other collections. Books contained only-copy-extant books and rare classics since the Song, Yuan, Ming, and Qing Dynasties. Calligraphy works and paintings contained valuable works of celebrities and famous doctors from the above-mentioned periods. Other collections contained stoneware, copper ware, porcelain, lacquerware, ivories, carvings (bamboo carvings and wood carvings), silk and clay sculptures.

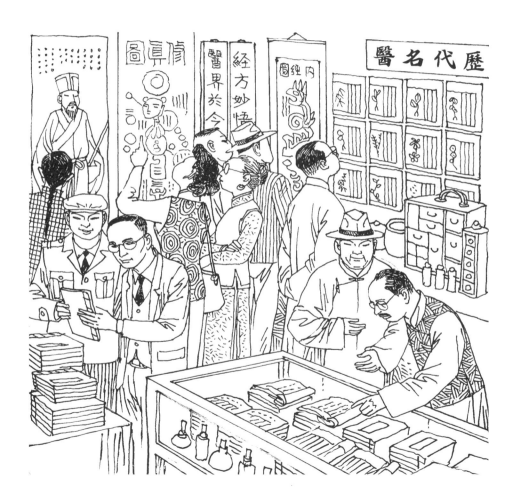

24 王吉民积极搜集医史文物，不少会员慷慨捐赠，先后征集到明清时期中药瓶、制药工具等，尤其珍贵的是前文提及的清代乾隆针灸铜人。其他还有晋代越窑青瓷"四耳药壶"、明代李濂《医史》、《本草纲目》的英文与法文节译本、清代医家书画、医学院校毕业证书、医学杂志及照片等。在王吉民的呼吁和各方支持下，博物馆藏品不断丰富。

Wang Jimin actively collected Chinese medical history relics, and many members of the museum generously donated their personal collections, including Chinese medicine bottles and pharmaceutical tools from the Ming and Qing Dynasties. Among them, the especially precious one was an acupuncture cooper figure dating back to the Qianlong Period of the Qing Dynasty. Other relics included "medicine pot with four handles" (blue porcelain of Yue Kiln in the Jin Dynasty), the *Medical History* (*Yi Shi*) written by Li Lian in the Ming Dynasty, the English and French translations of the *Compendium of Materia Medica*, calligraphy works and paintings by doctors in the Qing Dynasty, graduation certificates of medical schools, medical magazines and photos, etc.

Over the years, the museum's collection has grown steadily, thanks to Wang Jimin's impassioned appeals and the support garnered from various quarters.

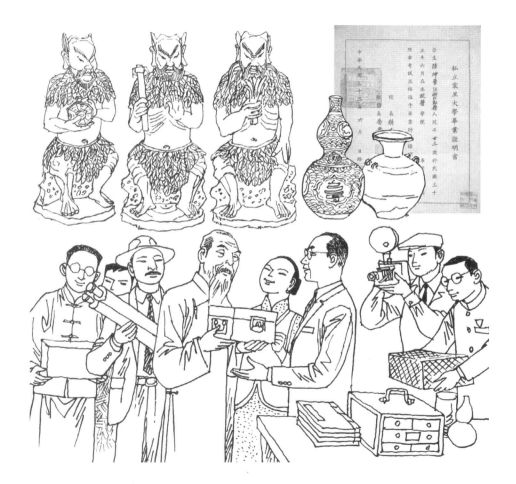

25 1954 年 2 月 19～28 日，李时珍文献展览会在中华医学会上海分会大礼堂举行，由中华医学会上海分会、中国药学会上海分会及中华医学会上海分会医史学会三个团体合办，专为会员展出。所展文物分为 5 类，分别是画像图表、传记论文、《本草纲目》各种版本、《本草纲目》各国译本及其他相关文物。展品中不乏稀有珍品，如《本草纲目》金陵版、朝鲜米尔斯英译《本草纲目》原稿、伊博恩英译《本草纲目》木部遗稿。最有意义的，当属李时珍的故乡及墓碑照片，为前人所未发，意义非凡。

The Exhibition of Li Shizhen's Document was held in the auditorium of Shanghai Branch of Chinese Medical Association from February 19 to February 28, 1954. This member-exclusive exhibition was jointly organized by three Shanghai Branches respectively affiliated with Chinese Medical Association, Chinese Pharmaceutical Association and Chinese Medical Association of Medical History. The showcased relics were divided into five categories, encompassing portraits, charts, biographies, dissertations, different versions and foreign edition of *Compendium of Materia Medica* and other related relics. Notably, the exhibition featured several rarities, such as the Jin Ling edition of the *Compendium of Materia Medica*, its original manuscript translated by Mills of North Korea and its posthumous manuscript translated by Bernard Emms Read. The most meaningful relics are photos of Li Shizhen's hometown and tombstone, which had never been displayed before.

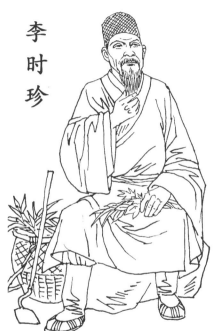

李时珍

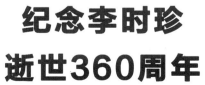

纪念李时珍
逝世360周年

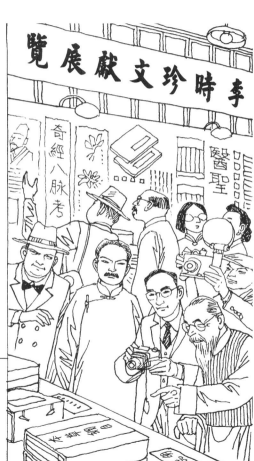

An Illustrated History of the Shanghai Museum of Traditional Chinese Medicine

26 1950 年，中华医学会总会由上海迁至北京，上海成立中华医学会上海分会，医史博物馆留在中华医学会上海分会。1956 年，中华医学会上海分会搬迁到国华大楼，被安排 1～3 楼用房。医史博物馆在 3 楼，分布有博物馆办公室 1 间，文物陈列室 5 间，资料室 1 大间，库房 1 间，整修、登记文物 1 间。藏品增至 2 229 件，陈列内容改为"医学史"和"李时珍文献"两个专题陈列。

In 1950, the Chinese Medical Association was relocated from Shanghai to Beijing, thus giving rise to the establishment of the Shanghai Branch of the Chinese Medical Association. Meanwhile, the Museum of Medical History remained in Shanghai. In 1956, the Shanghai Branch of the Chinese Medical Association moved to Guohua Building, where it occupied the first to third floors. The museum, situated on the third floor, comprised of 1 office, 5 exhibition rooms for relics, 1 large document room, 1 storage room, and 1 room for the repair and registration of cultural relics. Over time, the collection grew to encompass 2,229 pieces, leading to the division of the exhibition content into two sections: Medical History and Literature about Li Shizhen.

国华大楼

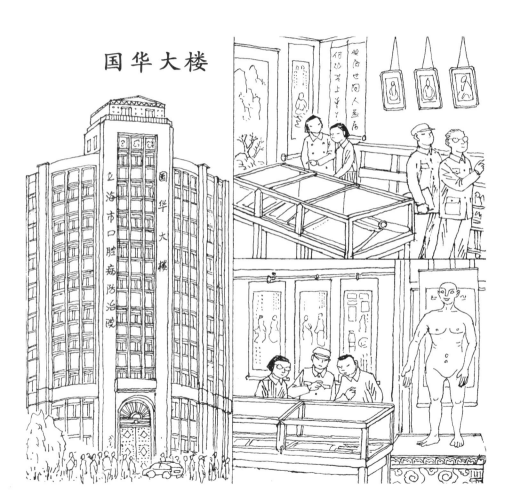

27 为征集收藏更多文物藏品，博物馆聘请了很多专家，朱孔阳便是其中的翘楚。王吉民和朱孔阳在抗日战争前已是挚友，1953年收藏家朱孔阳应王吉民之邀正式加入中华医学会医史博物馆工作，他以独到的文物鉴赏能力和丰厚的考据学方面知识，为文物征集工作提供了坚实的保障。

朱孔阳是当代著名社会活动家、金石书画家、文物鉴赏收藏家、医史学家，1978年被聘为上海文史馆馆员。早年投身于公益事业，同时对历代文物，既精鉴别，又富收藏。曾说："不只因为自己爱好，主要是为国家保存文物。"其发表的《历宋元明清二十余代重固名医世系考》，首次对江南何氏世医家传世系的起始年代进行考证，修正了之前何氏世医起于元代的说法。

To acquire a greater collection of cultural relics, the museum enlisted the expertise of numerous professionals, one of whom was Zhu Kongyang. Prior to the Chinese People's War of Resistance Against Japanese Aggression, Wang Jimin and Zhu Kongyang were already close friends. In 1953, Zhu was formally invited by Wang to join the Museum of Medical History of the Chinese Medical Association. With his extraordinary ability in identifying and appreciating cultural relics, as well as his vast knowledge on academic research, Zhu played an integral role in bolstering the museum's collection. Zhu Kongyang was widely recognized as a prominent contemporary social activist, an epigraphy and painting artist, a collector of cultural relics, and a medical historian. In 1978, he was employed as a librarian at the Shanghai Museum of Classical Literature and History. During his early years, Zhu devoted himself to public welfare and cultivated a passion for appreciating and collecting cultural relics. He once stated, "(I engage in this pursuit) not only for personal interest but also to preserve our country's cultural heritage." His work, *Research on the Genealogy of More Than 20 Generations of Famous Doctors in Chonggu Town in the Song, Yuan, Ming, and Qing Dynasties* (*Li Song Yuan Ming Qing Er Shi Yyu Dai Chong Gu Ming Yi Shi Xi Kao*), served as the initial verification of the He family's origin in the regions south of the Yangtze River. Zhu extensively studied the medical tradition of the He family, revising the previous belief that their medical practice originated in the Yuan Dynasty.

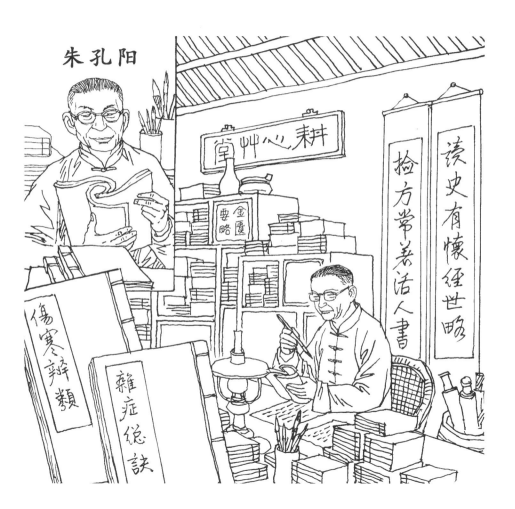

朱孔阳

耕心艸堂

金匱要略

拣方常善活人書

读史有懷經世略

傷寒辨類

雜症總訣

28 1939 年 11 月，《中华医学杂志》刊登徐灵胎撰写的《画眉泉记》。中华医学会医史博物馆于 1957 年向苏州市有关部门打听画眉泉旧址，都回复不知。

朱孔阳根据《画眉泉记》《乾隆苏州府志卷》《道光刊苏州府志》《宋平江城坊考》等古文献的记载线索，于 1958 年带领博物馆人员两度前往寻访，终于在江苏省苏州城外七子山东的"吴头山"，找到清代著名医家徐灵胎晚年隐居之地画眉泉旧址。继画眉泉访古以后，博物馆又陆续访得吴江徐氏的洄溪草堂、八坼的徐氏夫妇墓，亦成为医史考古的美谈。

In November 1939, the *Traditional Medical Journal of China* published the *Records of Huamei Spring* (*Hua Mei Quan Ji*) written by Xu Lingtai. In 1957, the museum reached out to relevant departments in Suzhou to inquire about the former location of the Huamei Spring, but unfortunately received no response.

Under the leadership of Zhu Kongyang, the museum staff embarked on two expeditions in 1958 to search for the Huamei Spring. They relied on clues found in ancient literature such as the *Records of Huamei Spring*, *Annuals of Suzhou During the Qianlong Period of Qing Dynasty* (*Qian Long Su Zhou Fu Zhi Juan*), *Annuals of Suzhou During the Daoguang Period of Qing Dynasty* (*Dao Guang Kan Su Zhou Fu Zhi*), and *Research on Pingjiang City in the Song Dynasty* (*Song Ping Jiang Cheng Fang Kao*). Eventually, they located the Huamei Spring on the eastern side of the Wutou Mountain, situated outside the urban areas of Suzhou and adjacent to the Qizi Mountain. This was the place where the renowned medical practitioner Xu Lingtai in the Qing Dynasty spent his later years in seclusion. The discovery of the Huamei Spring led the museum staff to subsequently uncover the sites of the Huixi Grass Hall of the Xu family in Wujiang district, as well as the grave of the Xu couple in Bache town. This became a notable story in the field of medical history archaeology.

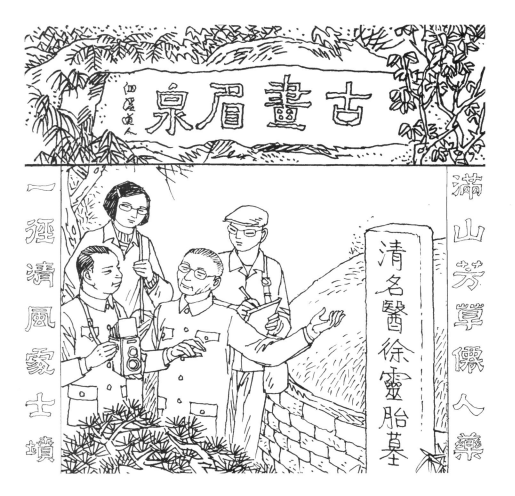

29 1959 年，博物馆由中华医学会改属于上海中医学院（现上海中医药大学），整体迁址于上海中医学院（零陵路 530 号）内。

博物馆在学院党委的直接领导下，得到长足发展，更明确了医史博物馆辅导教学的任务。博物馆陈列室配合中国医学史教学，委托上海美术设计公司重新布置，增加陈列文物名称、版面照片、示意图、文字说明等，并将李时珍文献展览会改名为李时珍纪念室。

重新布置后的上海中医学院医史博物馆由三部分组成，陈列室、李时珍纪念室和文献资料室。

In 1959, the Museum of Medical History, formerly under the auspices of the Chinese Medical Association, was transferred to the Shanghai College of Traditional Chinese Medicine (now Shanghai University of Traditional Chinese Medicine) at No.530 Lingling Road. Under the direct leadership of the college's Party Committee, our museum has made significant progress and further clarified its additional task of medical history teaching. To better assist with the teaching task, we have commissioned Shanghai Art-Designing Co. Ltd. to revamp the Exhibition Hall. This effort involved incorporating numerous supplementary elements such as detailed labels for the exhibits, layout photographs, diagrams and comprehensive explanatory notes. Furthermore, we have decided to rename the previous "Li Shizhen Literature Exhibition" to the more fitting designation of "Li Shizhen Memorial Hall". The rearranged museum consisted of three parts: Exhibition Hall, Li Shizhen Memorial Hall, and Documentation Room.

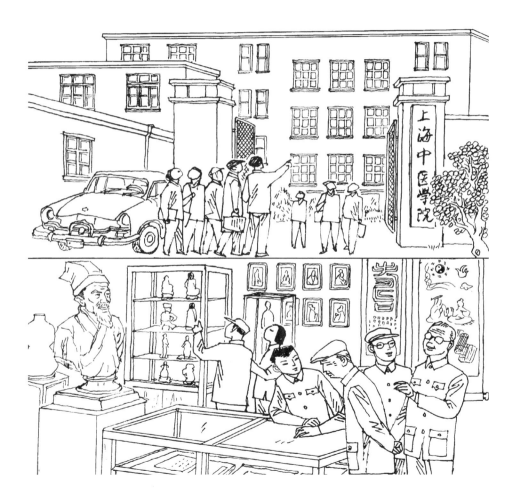

30 李约瑟博士，本名约瑟夫·尼达姆（Joseph Needham），是大家熟悉的《中国科学技术史》的作者。他曾 3 次（1946年、1964年、1984年）访问医史博物馆，为博物馆签名题词。

特别是 1964 年春天的这次，他看得非常仔细，记录非常认真，还把陈列的古代外科器械照了相。为了感谢他对中国医学史的重视和宣传，医史博物馆赠给他一张明代炼丹炉的照片和一册英文版的《中国针灸史话》。

Dr. Joseph Needham, renowned as the author of *Science and Civilization in China*, visited our museum 3 times (in 1946, 1964, and 1984) and wrote inscriptions for it. Especially during the visit in the spring of 1964, he paid meticulous attention and made comprehensive records. Additionally, he took photos of the exhibited ancient surgical instruments. To express sincere gratitude for his promotion of Chinese medical history, we presented him with a photo of a Ming Dynasty alchemy furnace and a copy of English edition of *The History of Chinese Acupuncture and Moxibustion* (*Zhong Guo Zhen Jiu Shi Hua*).

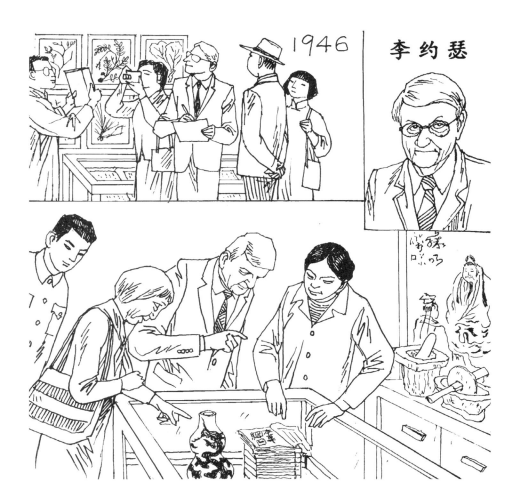

李约瑟

1946

31 1966 年以后，医史博物馆也与国家命运一样遭受磨难。全馆六人，不是赋闲、退休，就是被遣离，博物馆处于无人管理状况，文物险遭破坏。后来经过多方关心，从 1966 年 7 月起上海中医学院医史博物馆及时封馆，才使这座藏珍纳宝的博物馆，在被人冷落中得以保全。

After 1966, the Museum of Medical History endured immense hardship as the country went through ups and downs. At that time, the museum had mere six staff members, all of whom were either laid off, retired, or compelled to leave. Consequently, the museum was left unmanaged, posing a looming threat of damage to its precious cultural relics. Fortunately, with the support from all sides, the museum was promptly closed and protected since July 1966, thus these valuable cultural relics successfully survived.

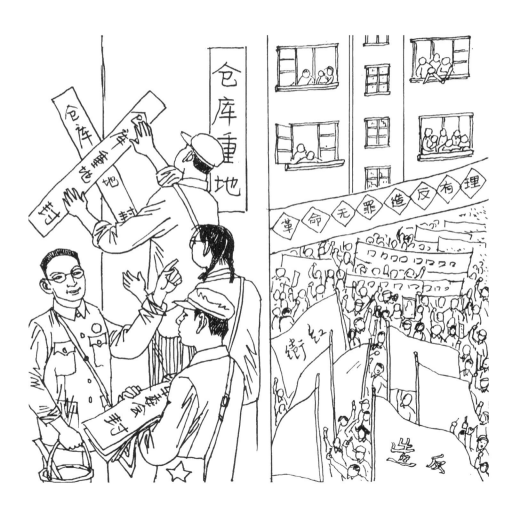

32 新中国成立后，医务人员遵照毛主席关于"古为今用，洋为中用""推陈出新"中西医结合的指示，积极发掘中医药学遗产。在群众性的推广中医针灸疗法的实践中，把针灸止痛和针灸治病的经验加以总结，大胆运用到外科手术上，成功开展了针刺麻醉。

1971 年 7 月 19 日，《人民日报》头版专栏刊登《毛主席无产阶级卫生路线和科研路线的伟大胜利——我国医务工作者和科学工作者创造成功针刺麻醉》。同年 11 月 25 日，《解放日报》和《文汇报》同时刊登由博物馆傅维康教授撰写的有关针刺麻醉专版，介绍针灸历史与针刺麻醉机制的探讨。此后，外文出版社选用《文汇报》刊登文章，翻译成英、法、德、日、俄、西班牙、朝鲜、越南文，收录在《中国的针刺麻醉》上述八种外文本中出版。

After the founding of the People's Republic of China, medical professionals adhered to Chairman Mao's instruction of "absorbing what is useful both in the past and in other parts of the world" and "rejecting what is useless and adding what is essentially your own", aiming to integrate TCM with Western medicine and develop our valuable national medical heritage. They practiced acupuncture and moxibustion extensively, summarized their experience of pain relief and treatment through acupuncture and moxibustion, and applied the experience to surgical procedures. With all those efforts, Chinese acupuncture anesthesia was finally created.

On July 19, 1971, the *People's Daily* published a featured article on its front page titled "*The Remarkable Achievement of Chairman Mao's Proletarian Healthcare and Scientific Research Guidance—Chinese Medical Workers and Scientific Researchers have Created Acupuncture Anesthesia.*" On November 25 of the same year, *Jiefang Daily* and *Wenhui Daily* published a special edition on Chinese acupuncture anesthesia, written by Professor Fu Weikang from our museum, which introduced the history of acupuncture and moxibustion as well as the mechanism of acupuncture anesthesia. Subsequently, the Foreign Languages Press selected the article published in *Wenhui Daily*, translated it into English, French, German, Japanese, Russian, Spanish, Korean and Vietnamese, and included it in the eight foreign languages' versions of *Chinese Acupuncture Anesthesia (Zhong Guo De Zhen Ci Ma Zui)*.

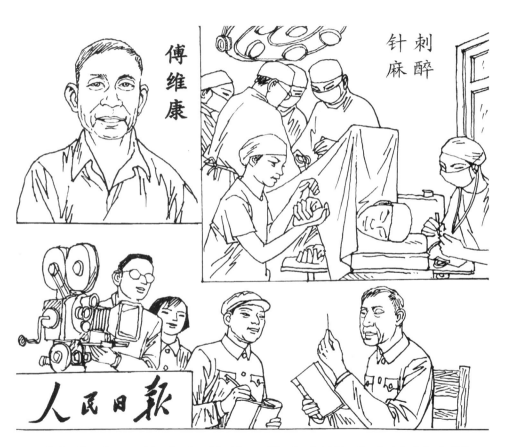

傅维康

针刺麻醉

我国医务工作者和科学工作者创造成功针刺麻醉

33 由于中国针刺麻醉的成功应用，在世界医学界引起很大反响。小小的银针发挥神奇疗效，为配合宣传针灸历史，上海科学教育电影制片厂拍摄《中国针刺麻醉》电影。

几经周折，终于在 1972 年初医史博物馆启封时科学教育电影厂摄制组实地踏看，只见展品尘封，积灰满地，但认为有拍摄价值。于是医史博物馆重新得到装修和布置，该馆人员除少数人以外，基本归队。尘垢洗尽，上海中医学院医史博物馆这面历史古镜又显真容，它为宣传祖国优秀的古代文化又立新功。

Chinese acupuncture anesthesia has attracted great attention from the world medical community for its high efficacy. To complement the promotion of the history of acupuncture and moxibustion, the Shanghai Science Education Film Studio filmed a movie called *Chinese Acupuncture Anesthesia* (*Zhong Guo Zhen Ci Ma Zui*).

After twists and turns, the Museum of Medical History was reopened in early 1972 and the film crew finally had the chance to visit it, only to find the exhibits covered in dust and dirt. However, the crew believed that it was valuable to film them. Therefore, the museum was renovated and redecorated, and most of the staff returned to work. Through a thorough cleansing, the Museum of Medical History of Shanghai College of Traditional Chinese Medicine revealed its historical splendor once more, once again making new contributions to the promotion of our esteemed ancient Chinese culture.

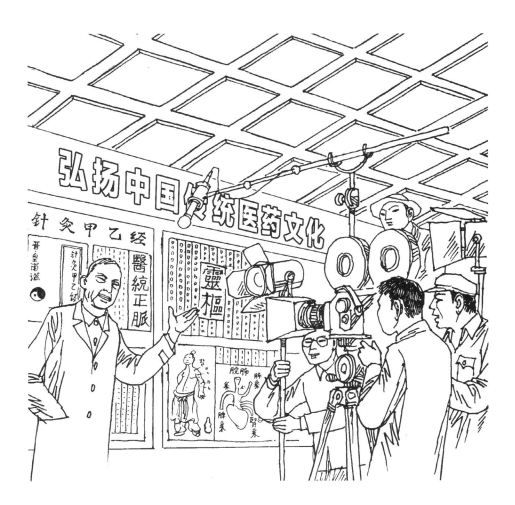

34 1973 年，上海中医学院新建 6 层的图书馆大楼，博物馆展陈在第三层。新展馆按通史顺序排列，分 12 块版面，26个专题，另有 12 个展览橱柜。让观众在观赏文物史迹过程中，得到艺术熏陶的同时，更领悟到中医药的形成和发展源远流长。

In 1973, Shanghai College of Traditional Chinese Medicine built a new six-story library with the museum on the third floor. The exhibits were chronologically arranged and categorized into 12 parts, 26 sections, and 12 display cases. It encouraged visitors to go deeper into the profound history of TCM while appreciating the artistic charm of these cultural relics.

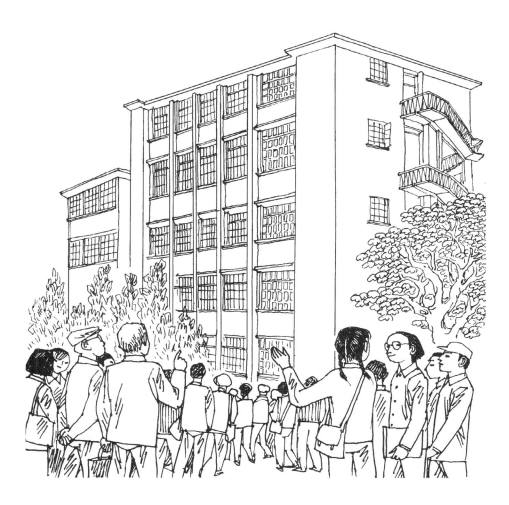

35 1975 年初冬，联合国世界卫生组织副总干事兰波先生特地安排了半天时间参观医史博物馆，结束参观后说："我回到联合国后，一定建议访问中国的世界卫生组织的代表也到这里来参观。"1978 年，兰波先生再度来到医史博物馆，并陪同尼日利亚、塞拉利昂、索马里、博茨瓦纳、卢旺达等国家的卫生部部长一起参观。此后，参加世界卫生组织传统医学考察团的40 多个国家的代表也先后三次前来参观医史博物馆。

In the early winter of 1975, Mr. Rambo, Deputy Director-General of the World Health Organization (WHO), made a half-day visit to the Museum of Medical History. "After I return to the United Nations, I will definitely recommend the representatives of WHO to visit this place when they come to China," he said. During his second visit in 1978, Mr. Rambo accompanied the health ministers of Nigeria, Sierra Leone, Somalia, Botswana, Rwanda and other countries to the museum. From then on, representatives of WHO traditional medicine delegation from more than 40 countries have visited the museum three times.

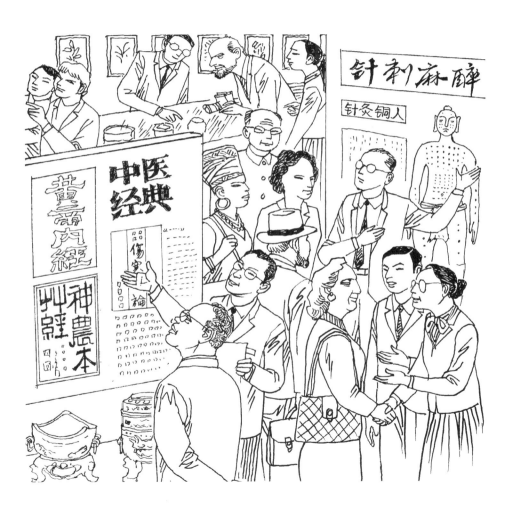

36 贾福华，1936年考入中国医学院学习，1937年因
"八一三"事变学业中缀，肄业后复从名医丁济万深造。于1947
年应儿科名家徐小圃传人王玉润先生之邀，进王家诊所，专业
儿科，仁术精进，声誉鹊起。

　　1956年进上海中医学院从事医史博物馆和医史教学工作，
1960年任医史博物馆副馆长，1978年任馆长。其间，笔耕不辍，
相继编写《中国医学史略》《医学杂文》《临床经验片断》等。

Jia Fuhua was admitted to the Chinese Medical College in 1936. However, he dropped out of school in 1937 due to the August 13th Incident, and followed the famous doctor Ding Jiwan for further study. In 1947, he was invited by Wang Yurun, a descendant of the famous pediatrician Xu Xiaopu, to work in the Wang's Clinic and became a professional and reputable pediatrician. In 1956, he started to work in the museum and teach medical history in Shanghai College of Traditional Chinese Medicine. He became the deputy curator of the Museum of Medical History in 1960 and the curator in 1978. Throughout this period, Jia remained committed to scholarly endeavors and authored several works, including *Chinese Medical History* (*Zhong Guo Yi Xue Shi Lyue*), *Medical Essays* (*Yi Xue Za Wen*) and *Fragments of Clinical Experience* (*Lin Chuang Jing Yan Pian Duan*).

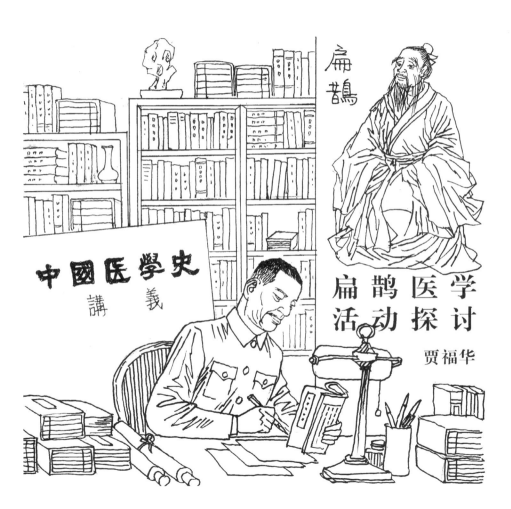

中國医學史
講義

扁鵲

扁鵲医学
活动探讨

贾福华

An Illustrated History of the Shanghai Museum of Traditional Chinese Medicine

37 1979 年 10 月，中国自然科学博物馆学会筹备工作会议在江苏南通举行。1980 年 12 月，中国自然科学博物馆学会在北京举行正式成立大会，上海中医学院医史博物馆成为该学会的团体会员，傅维康被选为该学会理事。1982 年 2 月，中国博物馆协会在北京举行成立大会，上海中医学院医史博物馆成为该协会的团体会员。

In October 1979, the preparatory meeting for the establishment of Chinese Association of Natural Science Museums was held in Nantong, Jiangsu Province. Subsequently, in December 1980, the association held its official founding meeting in Beijing. Museum of Medical History of Shanghai College of Traditional Chinese Medicine became a member of the association, whose director was Fu Weikang. In February 1982, the founding conference of the Chinese Museums Association was held in Beijing and the Museum of Medical History of Shanghai College of Traditional Chinese Medicine was selected as one of its members.

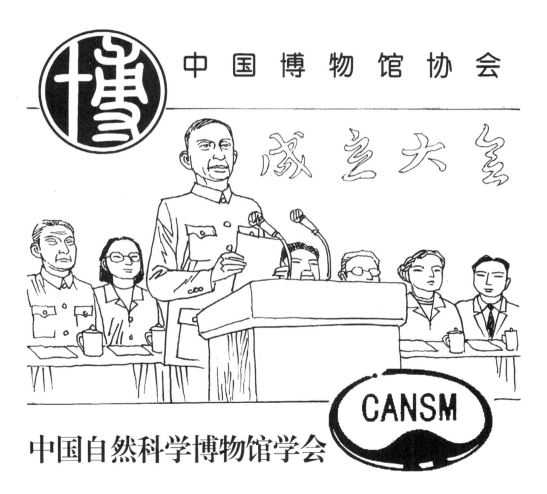

38 1987 年 9 月下旬，医史博物馆收到上海市电影局公函与电话，要求协助澳大利亚电影委员会（经中国文化部批准）拍摄介绍中国科技史的文化教育纪录片《萨那都之路》的若干中国医学史内容，傅维康馆长接受该纪录片摄制组采访后，陪同参观博物馆并对陈列文物讲解介绍，该摄制组选拍了一部分陈列室空间、文物和展出。

In late September 1987, the museum received a request from the Shanghai Film Administration to assist the Australian Film Commission (approved by the Ministry of Culture of the People's Republic of China) in filming Chinese medical history for the documentary *The Road to Sana'a*. Following the interview, Fu Weikang personally accompanied the crew to the museum and introduced cultural relics on display. During this period, they captured footage of the exhibition halls, cultural relics and exhibitions.

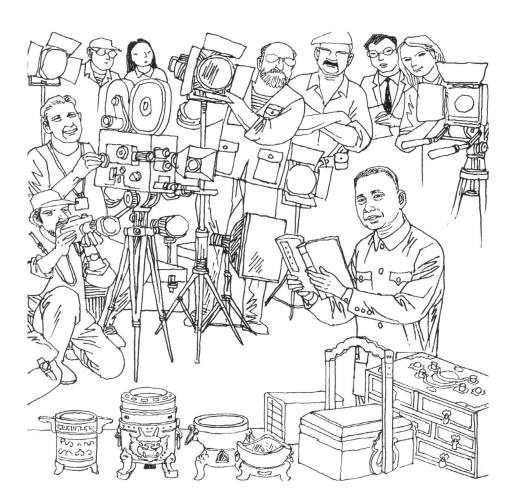

39 1988 年 7 月，医史博物馆建馆 50 周年，举行了隆重的系列庆祝活动。时任卫生部副部长、国家中医药管理局局长胡熙明题词"收集整理医史文物是振奋民族精神之大业"。国学家、科技史学家胡道静，上海博物馆馆长马承源，医史学家李经纬、程之范等为医史博物馆 50 周年题词。科技史学家李约瑟、医史学家文树德博士也发来了贺信。博物馆设计制作了 50 周年铜质圆形纪念章，一面图案为镇馆之宝针灸铜人；另一面图案为馆藏明黑釉葫芦瓶，周边设计 50 个圆点，一是代表药丸，二是表示医史博物馆建馆 50 周年。1988 年时值明代医家李时珍诞辰 470 周年，博物馆委托美术设计师彭天皿设计制作李时珍铜质纪念章。

The museum celebrated its 50th anniversary in 1988 and a series of celebrations were held in July. Hu Ximing, the vice minister of the Ministry of Health and director of the National Administration of Traditional Chinese Medicine, inscribed "Collecting and collating medical history and cultural relics is a great cause to uplift the national spirit". The anniversary was inscribed by Hu Daojing, a sinologist and historian of science and technology, Ma Chengyuan, director of the Shanghai Museum, as well as Li Jingwei and Cheng Zhifan, medical historians. In addition, Dr. Joseph Needham, historian of science and technology, and Dr. Paul Unschuld, historian of medicine, wrote congratulatory letters. The museum designed and produced a bronze commemorative medal to celebrate its 50th anniversary. One side of the medal features the acupuncture copper figure, symbolizing the most precious artifact of the museum. On the other side, there is a depiction of a black-glazed gourd-shaped bottle from the museum's collection, with 50 surrounding dots representing both medicinal pills and the 50th anniversary of the establishment of the museum. In 1988, commemorating the 470th birth anniversary of the renowned Ming Dynasty physician Li Shizhen, the museum commissioned the artistic designer Peng Tianmin to create a bronze medal in memory of him.

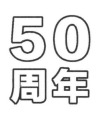

50周年

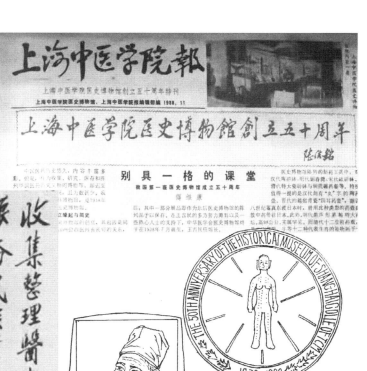

上海中医学院报

上海中医学院医史博物馆创立五十周年特刊
上海中医学院医史博物馆、上海中医学院报编辑部编 1988.11

上海中医学院医史博物馆創立五十周年

别具一格的课堂
我国第一座医史博物馆成立五十周年
傅维康

收集整理医史文物是
稜奋民族精神之大業

祝贺上海中医学院医史博物館創立五十周年

胡熙明
一九八八年十月

李時珍 1518-1593

THE 50TH ANNIVERSARY OF THE HISTORICAL MUSEUM OF SHANGHAI COLLEGE OF TCM
1938-1988

纪念章

40 根据王吉民创办博物馆的三个主要目的：① 搜集历代医史文物，"妥为保存，以免散失"，使"国粹不致外流"。② 将所收藏之文物，"供学者研究，藉以考察医学之变迁，治疗之演进"。③ "对学生为有效之教授方法，对民众可作宣传医药常识之利器"。博物馆长期坚持把科研工作放在十分重要的地位，历任馆长身体力行，带头进行科学研究，取得了一批重要成果。先后出版了《中文医史文献索引》《中国医学外文著述书目》《中国医史外文文献索引》《针灸文献索引》《中药学史》《针灸推拿学史》等，博物馆逐步形成一支中医文史学科群队伍，成为一个中国医学史研究的基地。随着社会对博物馆职能要求的提高，博物馆还注重将研究成果与教育、科学普及相结合。先后出版《上海中医药博物馆馆藏珍品》、《中医名家的故事》（视频）、《小学生中医药传统文化教育系列》、《闻香识本草》（视频）等。

In regards to the establishment of the museum, Wang Jimin had three main purposes: ① To collect the historical relics of medicine spanning the past dynasties. In so doing, "the quintessence of Chinese culture is properly preserved or it would be at risk of being lost". ② To make the cultural relics in the collection accessible to scholars for the purpose of studying the changes in medicine and the evolution of treatments. ③ "To not only provide an effective teaching method for students, but also serve as a valuable platform for promoting public awareness of medical knowledge". The museum has always put scientific research as a top priority. All curator has taken the lead in devoting themselves to scientific research, achieving tremendous progress. Many works were successively published, like *Index of Chinese Medical History Literature (Zhong Wen Yi Shi Wen Xian Suo Yin)*, *Bibliography of Foreign Literature on Chinese Medicine (Zhong Guo Yi Xue Wai Wen Zhu Shu Shu Mu)*, *Index of Foreign Literature on Chinese Medical History (Zhong Guo Yi Shi Wai Wen Wen Xian Suo Yin)*, *Index of Acupuncture and Moxibustion Literature (Zhen Jiu Wen Xian Suo Yin)*, *History of Chinese Materia Medica (Zhong Yao Xue Shi)*, *History of Acupuncture and Tuina (Zhen Jiu Tui Na Xue Shi)*, etc. Thanks to these efforts, the museum comes to be a base for research on the history of Chinese medicine with a team specialized in the cultural history of Chinese medicine. As societal expectations for the museum's functions have increased, the museum also focused on integrating research achievements with education and popular science. Publications such as *Treasures from the Collection of the Shanghai Museum of Traditional Chinese Medicine* (*Shang Hai Zhong Yi Yao Bo Wu Guan Guan Cang Zhen Pin*), *Stories of Famous Traditional Chinese Medicine Experts* (*Zhong Yi Ming Jia De Gu Shi*) (video), *Elementary School Students' Series on Traditional Chinese Medicine and Cultural Education* (*Xiao Xue Sheng Zhong Yi Yao Chuan Tong Wen Hua Jiao Yu Xi Lie*) and *Recognizing Medicinal Herbs by Their Fragrance* (*Wen Xiang Shi Ben Cao*) (video) have been released.

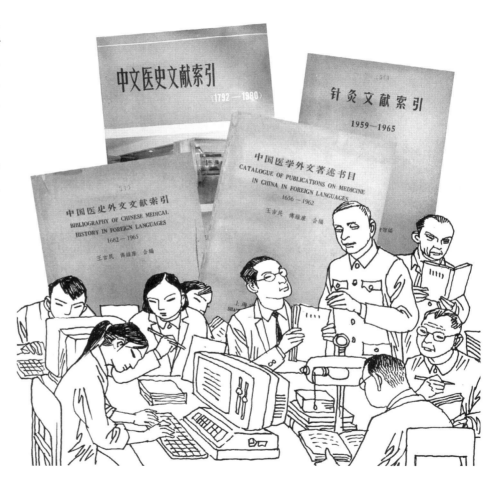

41 由博物馆傅维康教授和四川大学博物馆陈德福发起、组织的全国第一个高校博物馆学术团体——中国博物馆协会高等学校博物馆专业委员会于1994年成立，傅维康教授当选首届主任委员。中国博物馆协会高等学校博物馆专业委员会成立之后，在业界取得了广泛的影响。之后，吴鸿洲馆长继任主任委员和名誉主任委员。

In 1994, Higher Education Museums Special Committee of the Chinese Museums Association, the first national academic group in the field of higher education museums in China, was initiated and organized by Curator Fu Weikang of our museum and Chen Defu of Sichuan University Museum. Fu Weikang was elected as the inaugural chairman of the committee. Subsequently, Curator Wu Hongzhou succeeded as the chairman and honorary chairman of the committee. The committee gained widespread influence in the field since its establishment.

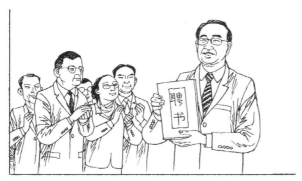

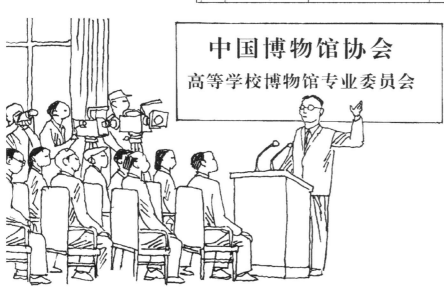

中国博物馆协会
高等学校博物馆专业委员会

42 1998 年 5 月初，上海中医药大学医史博物馆恢复属学校和中华医学会双重领导，以学校为主。在 5 月 12 日，中华医学会 / 上海中医药大学医史博物馆 60 年庆典暨学术研讨会上举行了揭牌仪式。

In early May 1998, the museum restored the dual leadership of the Shanghai University of Traditional Chinese Medicine as well as the Chinese Medical Association, and was mainly governed by the university. On May 12, the opening ceremony was held at the 60th anniversary celebration and symposium of the Museum of Medical History of Shanghai University of Traditional Chinese Medicine / Chinese Medical Association.

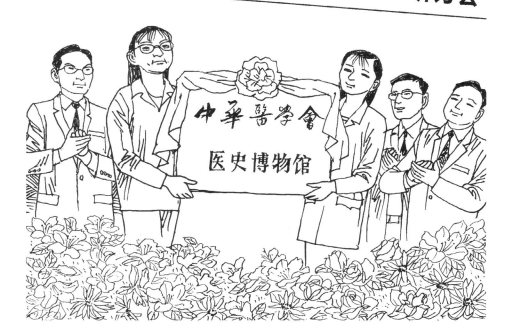

中华医学会　上海中医药大学
医史博物馆六十周年庆典暨学术研讨会

中華醫學會
医史博物馆

43 在各兄弟省市文物管理委员会、博物馆的大力协助和支持下，馆藏文物品种越来越丰富。上海市文物管理委员会曾支援了大批医史文物，如宋八卦星月纹铜串铃，明獬豸铜熏、炼丹铜炉，清药杵臼、八角铜手炉、长方脚炉等。之后，上海博物馆还调拨了 6 000 年前的井圈，并借展明代文徵明所写有关针灸治病内容的墓碑等。北京自然博物馆支援新石器时代的砭石，陕西省博物馆提供秦代下水道管和汉代鎏金铜熏炉等文物，山东省博物馆赠送石质按摩器，中国中医研究院药物研究所支援马王堆出土药物——桂皮、花椒、茅香，苏州市博物馆赠送骨针和云母片，福建省博物馆赠送宋代水银，南京市文物管理委员调拨晋代丹丸，泉州海外交通史博物馆调拨宋代药物——木香、沉香等，故宫博物院调拨一批文物，其中有"清御制如意金黄散"药方和"清御制平安丹"药方。这些都是医药文物珍品。

Supported by the management committees of cultural relics and museums from other provinces and cities, more varieties of cultural relics enriched the museum's collection. The Shanghai Management Committee of Cultural Relics offered a large number of medical historical relics, embracing the eight-trigram copper bell in stars and moon pattern in the Song Dynasty, the brass Xie Zhi (a legendary divine beast) fumigator in the Ming Dynasty, the alchemy brass furnace in the Ming Dynasty, the medicine mortar with pestle in the Qing Dynasty, the octagonal brass hand warmer in the Qing Dynasty, and the square foot warmer furnace in the Qing Dynasty. Later, the Shanghai Museum allocated a 6,000-year-old well loop. In addition to that, tombstones with inscriptions on acupuncture treatment by Wen Zhengming in the Ming Dynasty were loaned and displayed by the Shanghai Museum.

The Beijing Natural History Museum provided Bian-stones from the Neolithic Age, while Shaanxi Provincial Museum supplied artifacts such as the sewer pipe in the Qin Dynasty and the gold-gilded copper fumigator in the Han Dynasty. The Shandong Museum presented a stone massager. The Institute of Chinese Materia Medica, China Academy of Chinese Medical Science, donated unearthed herbal medicine including Cinnamon Bark (Cinnamoni Cortex), Pricklyash Peel (Pericarpium Zanthoxyli), and Sweet Grass (Hierochloe Odorata). The Suzhou Museum offered bone needles and mica tablets. The Fujian Museum gave the mercury of the Song Dynasty. The Nanjing Cultural Relics Administration Committee transferred the Dan pills of the Jin Dynasty. The Quanzhou Maritime Museum allocated medicines of the Song Dynasty encompassing Costus Root (Radix Aucklandiae), Eaglewood (Lignum Aquilariae Resinatum), etc. The Palace Museum allocated a number of cultural relics, containing the prescription of "Imperial Wishful Golden Powder of the Qing Dynasty (Qing Yyu Zhi Ru Yi Jin Huang San)" and the prescription of "Imperial Peace Pill of the Qing Dynasty (Qing Yyu Zhi Ping An Dan)". All of them are valuable medical relics.

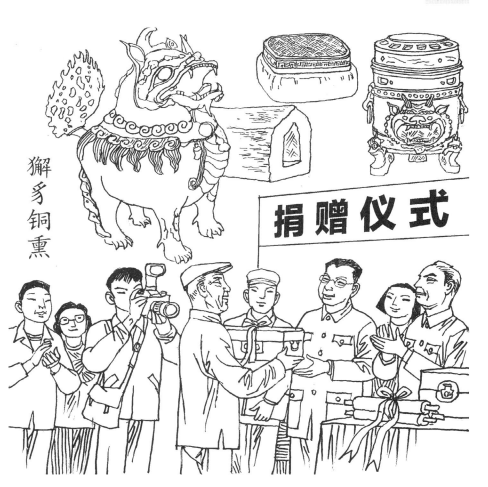

獬豸铜熏

捐赠仪式

44 个人捐赠的文物品种范围也十分广泛，有青铜器、瓷器、竹木器、象牙、骨器、玉器、画像、塑像、书画手迹等。如有张骧云膏方处方、脉案，抗日战争时期傅连暲木药箱，陈筱宝、石筱山、程门雪处方，吴昌硕行书七言五尺，何鸿舫、桂复隶书对联等。其中，1986年在上海中医学院名誉院长王玉润教授和沈家麒教授访美期间，旅美著名中国古董、古画鉴定家，远东艺术公司总裁曹仲英先生把自己珍藏的一幅清代晚期第一流的岭南派大师苏仁山（长春）的画，送给了博物馆。画面上是两位秦代名医——医和、医缓的图像。此画原为孙中山先生的医生——李岂劳博士所收藏，画上还有岭南派大画家高剑父的题跋。这幅画无论从艺术欣赏价值或收藏价值来说，都是非常宝贵的。馆藏的许多医史文献资料也是各界人士捐赠的。

In addition to the aforementioned relics, the museum received a wide range of cultural relics donated by individuals. These donations encompass bronze ware, porcelain ware, bamboo and woodware, ivory ware, bone ware, jade ware, portraits, statues, calligraphy works, and paintings, etc.

For example, notable items include the prescriptions and pulse cases of Zhang Xiangyun, the wooden medical kit that Fu Lianzhang carried with him during the Chinese People's War of Resistance Against Japanese Aggression, prescriptions written by Chen Xiaobao, Shi Xiaoshan, and Cheng Menxue, the seven-character couplet of five chi (about 167 cm) by Wu Changshuo, and a couplet written in clerical script by He Hongfang and Gui Fu, etc.

Among them, there is a painting by Su Renshan (also called Changchun), a superior master of the Lingnan School in the late Qing Dynasty. It was treasured by Mr. Cao Zhongying, a well-known Chinese antique and ancient painting appraiser and president of Far Eastern Art Company, who was sojourning in America. He gave the painting to the museum when Professor Wang Yurun and Professor Shen Jiaqi, Honorary Deans of Shanghai College of Traditional Chinese Medicine, visited the United States in 1986.

On the painting there are portraits of two eminent doctors of the Qin Dynasty, Yi He and Yi Huan. It was initially collected by Dr. Li Qilao, Sun Yat-sen's doctor. Besides, the painting was inscribed by Gao Jianfu, a great painter of the Lingnan School. Therefore, it is undoubtedly of great value in both art appreciation and collection. Moreover, a substantial portion of the medical history documents in the collection was also donated by people from all walks of life.

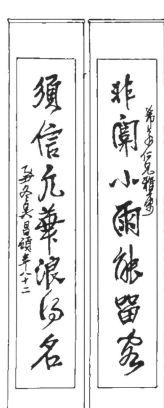

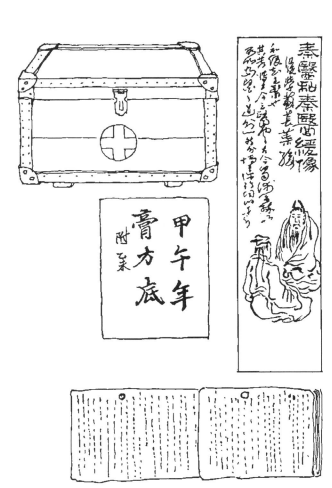

45 这一时期文物藏品征集不仅得到学校经费的支持，还得到很多专家的帮助。他们拥有丰厚的考据学方面知识和独到的文物鉴赏能力，为文物征集工作提供了坚实的保障。博物馆从文物商店、古玩市场等购买了明高县医学记铜印、唐黄釉脉枕、明镂空熏球、明炼丹炉、明木瓢（托钵）、明檀香切药刀、清青花药瓶等文物，进一步丰富了馆藏。

During this period, the collection of cultural relics not only received support from school funding but also garnered assistance from numerous experts. These experts possess rich knowledge in textual research and are able to appreciate cultural relics insightfully, providing solid support for the collection of cultural relics. We purchased the copper seal of "Gao Xian Yi Xue Ji" (Gao County Administration of Medicine) in the Ming Dynasty, yellow glazed pulse pillow in the Tang Dynasty, hollowed copper ball fumigator in the Ming Dynasty, alchemy furnace in the Ming Dynasty, wooden ladle in the Ming Dynasty, sandalwood medicine cutter in the Ming Dynasty, and blue-and-white medicine bottle in the Qing Dynasty from cultural relics shops and antique markets, further enriching the collection.

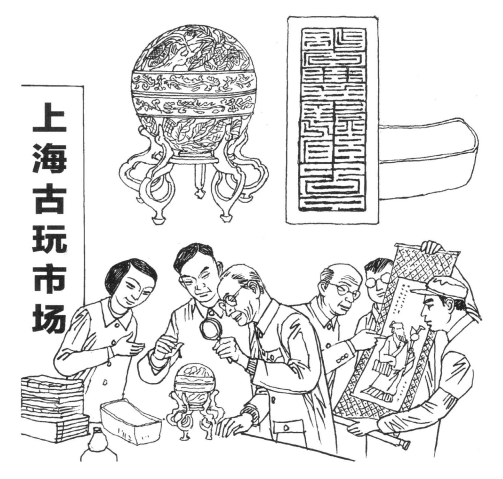

上海古玩市场

46 2003 年，实施上海市高校布局调整规划，上海中医药大学整体搬迁至浦东张江高科技园区，利用此机会，为博物馆单独建造了单体 3 层大楼，并将其布局在校园的最佳位置。全馆建筑面积 6 314 m²，其中第一、第二层为医史博物馆，第三层为中药标本馆、校史馆。

2003 年 10 月，上海中医药大学 / 中华医学会医史博物馆、中药标本室、党史校志编辑办公室，合并组建为上海中医药博物馆，同时保留上海中医药大学 / 中华医学会医史博物馆名称。2004 年 2 月 16～18 日，根据学校搬迁领导小组"精心组织，极端认真，细致周密，万无一失"的搬迁要求，医史博物馆、中药标本陈列室从零陵路校区平安搬迁至新校区。

In 2003, as part of the Shanghai University Layout Adjustment Plan, Shanghai University of Traditional Chinese Medicine moved to Zhangjiang High Technology Park, Pudong New Area. Taking this opportunity, a separate 3 story building for the museum was built and arranged in the optimal location of the campus. The museum has a total floor area of 6,314 m². The first and second floors house the exhibition halls for medical history, while the third floor is designed to showcase TCM specimens and the school's history.

In October 2003, the Shanghai Museum of Traditional Chinese Medicine (Museum of Medical History of the Chinese Medical Association), the Exhibition Hall of Chinese Medicine Specimen, and the Office of Party History and School Journal were merged into the Shanghai Museum of Traditional Chinese Medicine. At the same time, the name of the Shanghai Museum of Traditional Chinese Medicine (Museum of Medical History of the Chinese Medical Association) was retained. From February 16 to 18 in 2004, following the guidelines set by the school relocation leadership group, which emphasized meticulous organization and thorough arrangement, the Museum of Medical History, and the Exhibition Hall of Chinese Medicine Specimen were safely relocated from the Lingling Road campus to the new campus.

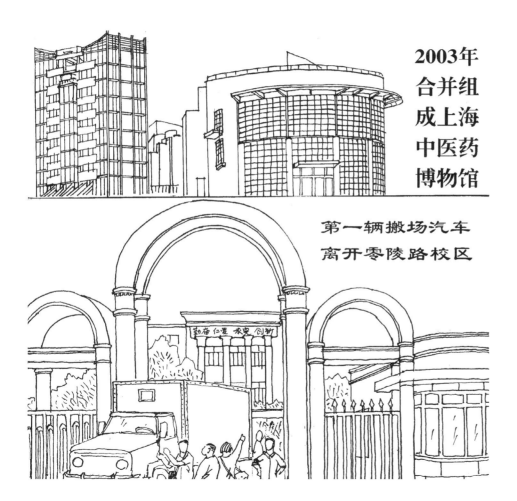

2003年
合并组
成上海
中医药
博物馆

第一辆搬场汽车
离开零陵路校区

An Illustrated History of the Shanghai Museum of Traditional Chinese Medicine

47 上海中医药博物馆组建前，仅有医史博物馆陈列室 240 m²，展示展品 1 214 件，以中国医学发展史为展示内容。上海中医药博物馆组建后，占地面积 2 200 m²，展览面积 4 300 m²。其中一楼医史综合馆介绍各个历史阶段中医药的突出成就和著名医家的主要活动，展示中医 5 000 年发展的基本脉络；二楼养生康复馆、针灸推拿馆、中医文化馆、中药方剂馆、中医科教馆，简要反映中医药在康复养生等各个领域的发展成就。一楼综合馆和二楼 5 个分馆展项展品 1 060 余件（套）。三楼中药标本陈列馆展品 1 500 多件；校史陈列馆陈列图片、实物 700 多件，扼要介绍并反映上海中医药大学自 1956 年创建以来的发展历程。全馆展项展品合计 3 200 余件。

Prior to the establishment of the Shanghai Museum of Traditional Chinese Medicine, there was only a single exhibition room in the Museum of Medical History. It covered an area of 240 m² with 1,214 items, primarily introducing the development of Chinese medicine. Now, the Shanghai Museum of Traditional Chinese Medicine has expanded to 2,200 m² with exhibition halls covering 4,300 m². Located on the first floor, the Comprehensive Hall of Medical History illustrates notable achievements of TCM throughout different historical periods. It also highlights major activities of famous TCM masters, and traces the development of TCM over a span of 5,000 years. The second floor comprises five exhibition halls: Health Preservation and Rehabilitation Museum, Acupuncture, Moxibustion and Tuina Hall, Traditional Chinese Medicine Culture Museum, Traditional Chinese Medicine Prescription Hall, and Traditional Chinese Medicine Education Hall. These halls showcase the achievements of TCM in fields such as rehabilitation and health preservation. The first and second floors exhibit more than 1,060 pieces (sets) of items. On the third floor, the Exhibition Hall of Chinese Medicine Specimen holds over 1,500 items on display. Besides, the Exhibition Hall of University History displays more than 700 pieces of pictures and other items. These briefly introduce the development of the Shanghai University of Traditional Chinese Medicine since its establishment in 1956. The total number of items on display amounts to 3,200.

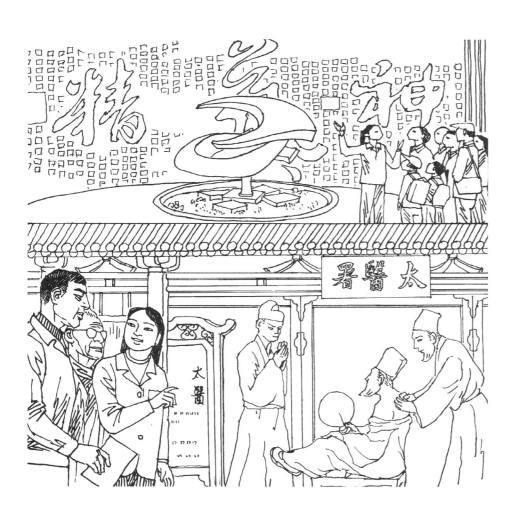

48 在新成立的上海中医药博物馆的三楼东侧是中药标本馆，有麝香、野山人参、冬虫夏草等名贵珍稀药材标本；矿物类精选标本；以根、茎、花、叶、果实、种子、全草入药的药材标本；中药炮制加工器械等展品，通过中药形态、功效、产地等介绍，向观众传播中药科学知识。许多在《本草纲目》中记录和描绘的中药材在这里以原药材、浸制标本、剥制标本、腊叶标本、药材饮片等形式进行展示，让人感到李时珍的这部东方药学巨典离我们并不遥远。腊叶标本、"道地药材"系列标本、中成药标本，主要来源于自采、征集和私人捐赠。历经几十年不断发展，已成为一个集教学、科研、对外交流和展示、科普宣传为一体的多功能中药标本展馆。

The newly built Shanghai Museum of Traditional Chinese Medicine houses the Exhibition Hall of Chinese Medicine Specimen on the east side of its third floor. There are rare specimens such as Musk (Moschus), wild Ginseng (Radix Ginseng), Chinese Caterpillar Fungus (Cordyceps) and more. Besides, there are a selection of mineral specimens and a batch of herbs whose roots, stems, flowers, leaves, fruits, seeds or whole plants can be used as medicine. Tools and machines applied to process medicinals are on display as well. By introducing the shape, function, and producing region, we can popularize TCM knowledge to the audience. Many herbs documented in the book *Compendium of Materia Medica* are exhibited in various forms, including raw materials, liquid preserved specimens, stripped specimens, pressed specimens, herbal pieces for decoction, etc. This approach brings us closer to the Chinese pharmaceutical classic written by Li Shizhen. These pressed specimens, specimens of genuine regional materia medica, and Chinese patent drugs are primarily collected from the museum, the public, or donations. After several decades of development, the Exhibition Hall of Chinese Medicine Specimen has an integrative function of teaching, scientific research, cultural exchange, and TCM popularization.

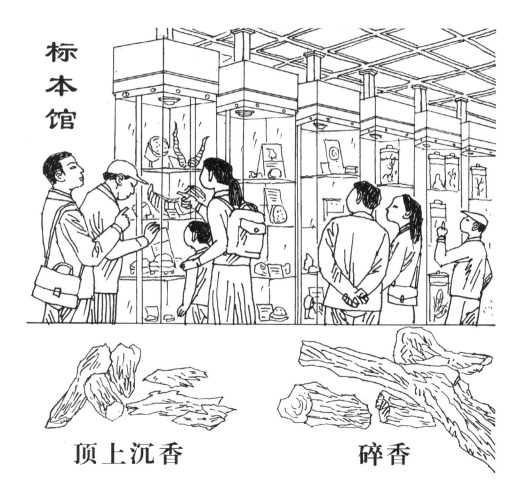

标本馆

顶上沉香　　碎香

49

2006 年，在上海市科学技术委员会的大力资助下，建造了"百草园·杏林苑"，整个园区被设计成八卦形与位于博物馆的"阴阳鱼"造型相对应。"杏林苑"栽种杏树 320 株，由学校教职员工和校友认养。每到农历二月杏花绽放时，全校师生都会不约而同地来此留影，是上海中医药大学的十大美景之一。"百草园"有下沉式广场、多媒体教室、暖房、人工小溪和喷水池等，种植 600 多种药用植物。

2020 年，在浦东新区政府及张江集团的大力支持下，百草园搬迁至吕家浜公共绿地，成为中医药文化园的"园中园"。将原来百草园的植物移栽至文化园内，并把李时珍塑像移至学校与百草园的入口处。同步在文化园内增加条石长廊、葫芦凳、藤蔓架、碎石小路等景观，做到层次起伏、错落有致、四季有景，开拓在区域内部小道，方便游客近距离观察草药。新百草园分 14 个主题园区，核心区域 7 200 m²，配备专业的标牌标识介绍，集专业性和观赏性于一体。

In 2006, with the sponsorship from the Science and Technology Commission of Shanghai Municipality, the Herb Garden and the Apricot Garden were built in the style of Eight Trigram matching the museum which is in the shape of yin-yang pair. In the Garden, there are 320 apricot trees adopted by faculty members and alumni. Each year, during the second month of the lunar calendar, the blooming apricot flowers attracts teachers and students to take photos here, for it is one of the top ten sceneries in the university. The Herb Garden is equipped with a sunken square, a multimedia classroom, a greenhouse, an artificial river, a fountain, etc. What's more, there are over 600 medicinal herbs.

In 2020, sponsored by the government of Pudong New Area and Zhangjiang Group, the Herb Garden was moved to Lyujiabang Public Greenland, where it became a part of the TCM Culture Garden. The herbs were transplanted to the new garden while the sculpture of Li Shizhen was relocated to the entrance of the Herb Garden to the university. Meanwhile, public facilities such as stone corridors, gourd stools, vine racks, gravel paths, and more were installed. All are arranged in a harmonious design, and the scenery varies with each season. The paths inside enable tourists to observe the herbs closely. The new garden consists of 14 themed areas with a central area of 7,200 m². It is equipped with introduction signages that embody medical knowledge and aesthetics.

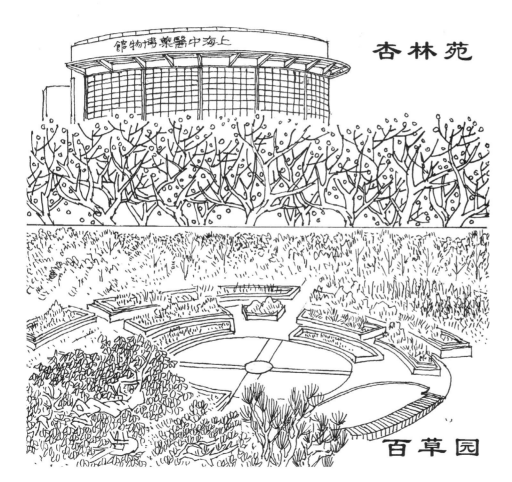

杏林苑

百草园

50 上海中医药博物馆建设项目被列为 2004 年度上海市科普实事工程项目。其展陈"中医药千年回想——中医药发展历程展"坚持"传统与现代结合、内涵与形式结合、借鉴与创新结合、中医与文化结合、中国古代哲学与中医学结合、中医学理论与临床成就结合",使学术性较强、比较枯燥的陈列内容变得生动活泼,通俗易懂,因此获上海市科学技术普及奖三等奖。上海中医药博物馆作为全国科普教育基地、全国中医药文化宣传教育基地,常年来为弘扬科学精神、宣传科学思想、推广科学方法、普及科学知识做了许多工作。出版的《中医名家的故事》作为"面向青少年的中医药系列科普读物"之一,获得 2019 年上海市科学技术普及奖一等奖。参与的"新冠肺炎中医药防控系列科普体系的创建与推广"项目获 2020 年上海市科学技术普及奖一等奖。参与的"中医药文化教育资源建设及推广——大中小学贯通融合的传承与创新教育实践"项目获 2022 年上海市教学成果奖特等奖。

In 2004, the construction project of the Shanghai Museum of Traditional Chinese Medicine was included in the Shanghai Science Popularization Program. Its exhibition *A Review of the Millennia's Development of TCM* sticks to "the integration of traditional and modern elements, content and form, borrowing and innovation, TCM and culture, Chinese ancient philosophy and traditional Chinese medicine, as well as TCM theory and clinical achievements". By this means, the dull academic exhibition was transformed into interesting and easily understandable experience. It, therefore, was granted the third prize of the Shanghai Science and Technology Award. The Shanghai Museum of Traditional Chinese Medicine serves as both an education base for national science popularization and a hub for promoting TCM culture. The museum has been dedicated to spreading the spirit, thoughts, methods, and knowledge of science. Its publication *Stories of Famous Traditional Chinese Medicine Practitioners* (*Zhong Yi Ming Jia De Gu Shi*) was recommended as a popular science reading for youngsters. It was also awarded the first prize of the 2019 Shanghai Science and Technology Award. The program *Establishment and Promotion of a Science Popularization System on COVID-19 Prevention and Control with Traditional Chinese Medicine* won the first prize of the 2022 Shanghai Science and Technology Award. Additionally, the program *Establishment and Promotion of TCM Culture Education Resource with Inheritance and Innovation Educational Practices for Undergraduates to Pupils* received the 2022 Shanghai Special Award of Teaching Achievement.

上海市科学技术奖励大会

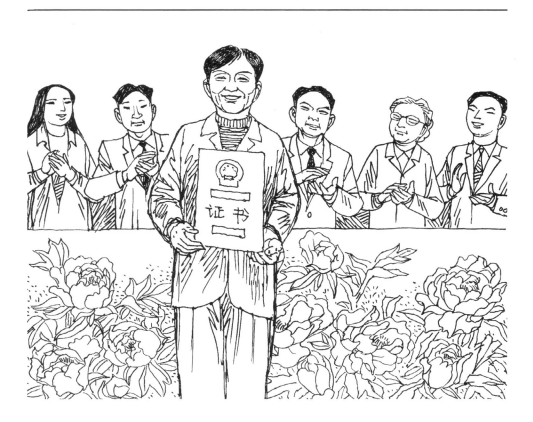

An Illustrated History of the Shanghai Museum of Traditional Chinese Medicine

51 博物馆致力于通过展览和各类主题活动宣传中医药知识，弘扬中医药文化，提高民众健康理念，促进民众健康生活，每年开展中医药主题活动 100 余场，开设各类讲座近 100 堂，形成"杏林科普"博物馆科普品牌活动和"岐黄博苑"博物馆学术品牌活动两大自主品牌。每年结合全国科普日、科技活动周、中国民俗传统文化节日等，以"请进来"和"送出去"多种方式，开展"灵丹妙药动手做""闻香识本草""国医节""迎新健身跑""小神农大赛"等多种竞赛、讲座和主题活动。同时，博物馆还充分利用大学生文化素质教育平台，不仅为医学生提供医史医德教育，还培养大学生志愿讲解员、开设"人文实践"课。

We are committed to promoting TCM knowledge and culture, as well as improving public health concepts and lifestyles through exhibitions and various theme activities. Annually, we host over 100 TCM activities and nearly 100 lectures. Two of our renowned events: the popular science event "TCM Popularization" and the academic event "TCM Seminar" have now become our icons. Every year, we organize competitions such as "Panaceas DIY", "Identifying Herbs by Smelling", "Chinese Medicine Day", "Running Workouts for Celebrating Chinese New Year", and "Competition of Little Shennong" on holidays like National Science Popularization Day, National Science and Technology Activity Week, and Traditional Chinese Folk Festivals. These activities take place either within the museum premises or by encouraging our staff to participate. Additionally, as part of our cultural education for college students, our goal is not only to provide medical students with education on medical history and medical ethics, but also to train undergraduate students to serve as volunteer commentators and engage in humanistic practices.

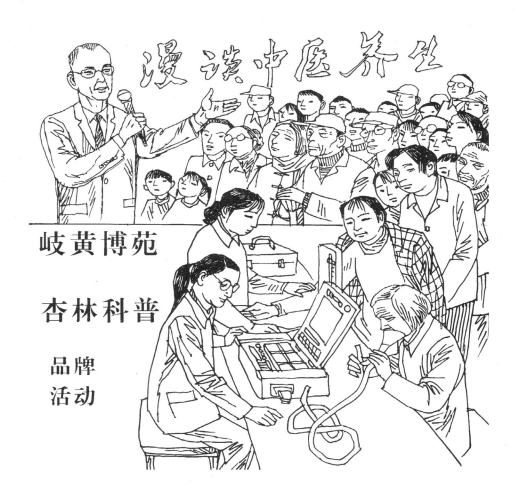

岐黄博苑

杏林科普

品牌
活动

An Illustrated History of the Shanghai Museum of Traditional Chinese Medicine

52 2016 年，博物馆完成了为期 9 个月的提升改造后，焕然一新的博物馆分为原始医疗活动、古代医卫遗存、历代医事管理、历代医学荟萃、养生文化撷英、近代海上中医、本草方剂鉴赏、当代岐黄新貌八个专题，反映了中医学在各个历史时期取得的主要成就。5 月 18 日，中华医学发展史陈列展暨第 40 个国际博物馆日"中医药文化景观进社区"研学活动启动仪式隆重举行。

In 2016, following a nine-month renovation, the new museum was divided into eight sections: Primitive Medical Practice, Preserved Artifacts in Ancient Health Care, Ancient Medical Practice Management, Historical Medical Collection, Ancient Chinese Culture on Life Nurturing, Modern Chinese Medicine in Shanghai, Appreciation of Herbal Prescriptions, and New Look of Contemporary Chinese Medicine. These sections showcase the major achievements of TCM throughout various historical periods. On May 18, various events took place, including the "Exhibition of the Development History of TCM," the opening ceremony of the 40th International Museum Day, and the academic activity on the "Chinese Medicine Cultural Landscape in the Community".

中华医学发展史陈列展

揭幕仪式

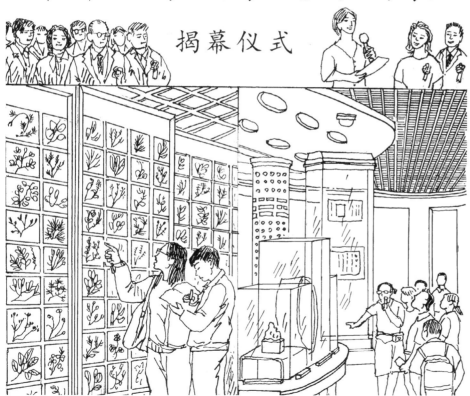

53 2018 年，中华医学会 / 上海中医药大学医史博物馆建馆 80 周年系列纪念活动隆重举行。自 2018 年新年伊始，博物馆开展了"迎新健身跑"、"第五届讲解比赛"、"新安医家墨迹展"、"闻香识药"科普活动和"国色天香医艺相融——汤兆基牡丹艺术展"等纪念活动。11 月，举办"岁月留珍——中华医学会 / 上海中医药大学医史博物馆建馆 80 周年回顾展"。11 月 14～16 日，召开中华医学会医史学分会第十五届第二次学术年会暨中华医学会 / 上海中医药大学医史博物馆建馆 80 周年研讨会。中华医学会党委书记苏志在开幕致辞中对博物馆建馆 80 周年表示热烈祝贺，就博物馆在医学会创办时期的文物收藏工作给予了高度评价。国医大师、全国名中医、中医院校老校长一行 22 人在上海中医药博物馆召开"中华医学会 / 上海中医药大学医史博物馆建馆 80 周年纪念活动——名医大师高端圆桌会议"。会议前，老专家们纷纷为博物馆建馆 80 周年纪念留下墨宝，国家级名老中医栗德林题词："国宝遗存，永放光彩。"甘肃中医学院原院长张士卿题诗一首："老树新枝生力强，杏林春暖硕果香，造福桑梓功德著，大美中医谱新章。"

In 2018, the Shanghai Museum of Traditional Chinese Medicine (Museum of Medical History of the Chinese Medical Association) celebrated its grand 80th anniversary with a series of commemorative activities. Throughout the year, memorial events were held, such as the "Running Workouts for Celebrating Chinese New Year", "The Fifth Commentator Competition", "Calligraphy Exhibition of Xin'an Physicians", "Identifying the Herbs by Smelling", and "Tang Zhaoji's Peony Painting Exhibition". In November, a retrospective of the Museum of Medical History's 80th Anniversary was organized to honor its establishment. From November 14 to 16, the Second Congress of the 15th Chinese Medical Association of Medical History was held, so as a Seminar on the 80th Anniversary of the museum. Su Zhi, the secretary of the Party Committee of the Chinese Medical Association, warmly congratulated the institution on its 80th anniversary and commended the efforts made in collecting relics during the association's founding period. A group of 22 esteemed experts, including TCM Masters, prominent TCM experts, and former presidents of TCM colleges, were invited to the Shanghai Museum of Traditional Chinese Medicine for the TCM Expert Summit, which served as an activity for the 80th anniversary celebration. Prior to the summit, the experts conveyed their sincere hopes and congratulations through their calligraphy. Notably, Li Delin, a prominent TCM expert, and Zhang Shiqing, the former Dean of Gansu College of

Traditional Chinese Medicine, inscribed special pieces in honor of the anniversary.

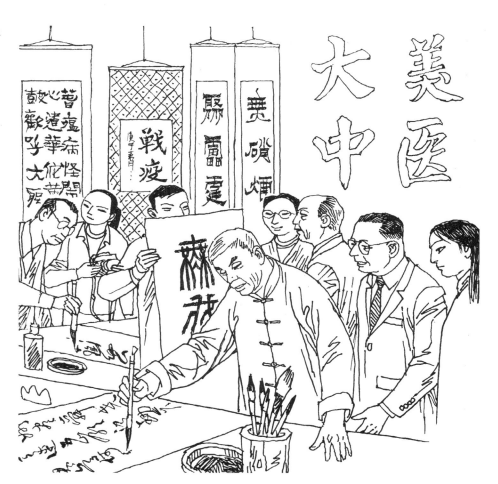

54 上海中医药博物馆作为中医药文化传播使者，先后到美国、英国、法国、比利时等 13 个国家举办中医药文化展。每个展览都配合了主题讲座、互动体验活动和民乐武术表演等，体现了"建立多形式、多层次、多维度的中医药国际传播方式，展示中医药的发展成就和成果，促进中医药更广泛地走向世界，服务人类健康"的宗旨。

The Shanghai Museum of Traditional Chinese Medicine, as a promoter of TCM culture, has successfully organized TCM cultural exhibitions in 13 countries, including the United States, the United Kingdom, France, and Belgium. Each exhibition featured thematic lectures, interactive experience activities, folk music, and martial arts performances. These exhibitions reflect our aim of establishing a diverse, comprehensive, and multidimensional international communication platform for TCM, revealing TCM's accomplishments and promoting its widespread adoption in the pursuit of human health.

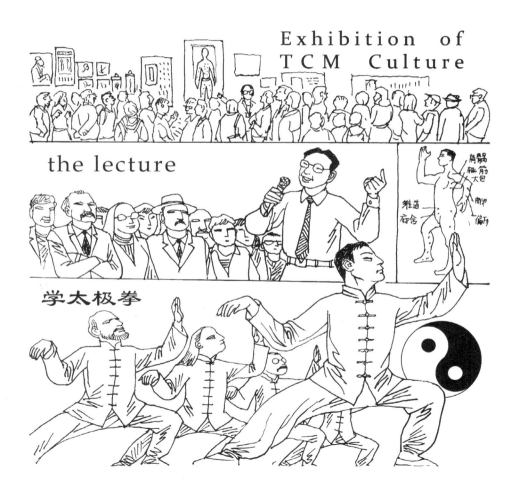

Exhibition of TCM Culture

the lecture

学太极拳

2020 年 6 月，上海交通大学—上海中医药大学全球中医药文化与创意研究中心挂牌仪式在上海中医药博物馆举行。研究中心致力于中医药文化的科普传播和大众推广，并针对中医药传统文化的传承与文化推广搭建一批文化传播平台，打造更多适合面向大众的中医药文化体验项目与文创产品，助力中医药文化的普及与传播。早在 1981 年博物馆就有文创设计，设计制作了铜质铸孙思邈像章。1982 年博物馆又以医史博物馆收藏的明黑釉葫芦瓶和明獬豸铜熏为图案，设计铸制两种铜质纪念章。1988 年设计制作铜质李时珍纪念章等。之后博物馆还设计五行棋、五行牌、博物馆图章、明信片、扇子、杯垫等各类中医药文创产品。中心成立后设计的时令中草药香囊，医缓医和图笔袋、环保袋，以及"灵兰"书签、生肖文件夹、中草药手账等一系列文创产品陆续"上线"，让传统中医药文化绽放出时尚的光彩。

Shanghai Jiao Tong University and Shanghai University of Traditional Chinese Medicine have collaboratively established the Global Cultural and Innovation Research Center for Traditional Chinese Medicine. The opening ceremony of this center took place at the Shanghai Museum of Traditional Chinese Medicine in June 2020. The center aims to promote TCM culture among the general public and facilitate the inheritance and dissemination of TCM culture through various means, such as establishing platforms for cultural communication, organizing TCM-experiencing programs, and creating TCM cultural products. In 1981, we designed and produced a bronze badge featuring Sun Simiao. Subsequently, in 1982, we cast two bronze badges inspired by the black-glazed gourd-shaped bottle and the brass Xie Zhi (a legendary divine beast) fumigator from the Ming Dynasty. Additionally, a bronze memorial medal of Li Shizhen was produced in 1988. Over time, we have designed more TCM products, including five-element chess and cards, museum stamps, postcards, fans, and mug mats. Following the establishment of the center, we introduced seasonal herbal sachets, pencil cases, eco-friendly bags, bookmarks, Chinese Zodiac clamps, and notebooks. These products effectively combine TCM culture with fashion trends.

全球中医药
文化与创意研究中心
成立仪式

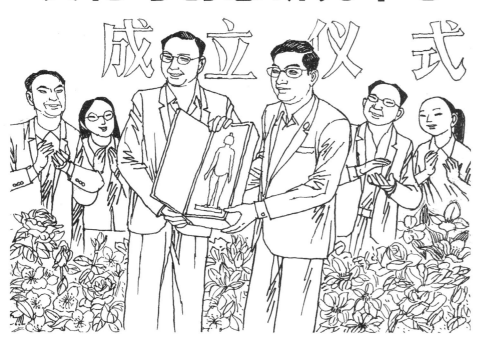

56 现今博物馆文物藏品已达到 14 590 件，征集的主要途径是接受捐赠和购买。随着文物博物馆事业的发展，博物馆也开始注重"为明天而收藏今天"。新型冠状病毒感染防治期间，博物馆第一时间发出征集公告，征集到"第四批国家中医医疗队（上海）队旗附医生签名"等数百件抗疫见证物。同时，博物馆通过捐赠、调拨、购买等方式不断丰富馆藏。如捐赠的藏品有：青海红十字医院院长张建青捐赠的马家窑文化陶器；郁慕馨（张伯讷遗孀）捐赠的张氏医案、处方及古琴；邵允明捐赠的吴昌硕题李霖斋诊室挂匾（木）；施维智捐赠的"特配"章及古书；许四海捐赠的手工紫砂壶；项斯玲夫妇捐赠的名家字画；林乾良捐赠的"春晖"名医书法。调拨的藏品有：上海科技馆调拨的中药标本云母等。使用专项征集经费购买有：唐云花鱼画；古八卦瓶；朱孔阳菊花图等。

Currently, the museum houses a collection of 14,590 cultural relics, primarily obtained through donations and purchases. As the museum expands, we come to realize the importance of "collecting the present for the future". During the COVID-19 pandemic, we promptly sent out notices to collect items that witnessed the fight against the pandemic and received hundreds of items, including the signature flag of the fourth batch of the national TCM Team (Shanghai). Simultaneously, we diligently seek to enrich our collection through donations, allocations, and purchases. For example, we have received donations of Majiayao Potteries from Zhang Jianqing, director of the Qinghai Red Cross Hospital, as well as medical records, prescriptions, and a guqin (a seven-stringed plucked instrument) belonging to Zhang Bone, generously provided by Mrs. Yu Muxin (Zhang Bone's wife). Moreover, we have received a medical practice plaque bestowed to Li Linzhai by Wu Changshuo from Mr. Shao Yunming, a special seal and ancient books from Mr. Shi Weizhi, handmade purple clay pots from Mr. Xu Sihai, precious calligraphies and paintings from the Xiang Silin family, as well as a piece of calligraphy on spring from Mr. Lin Qianliang. Notably, some of our items were allocated, including Mica specimens from the Shanghai Science and Technology Museum. Additionally, we have made purchases with special funds for collection, such as acquiring flower and fish paintings by Tang Yun, an ancient eight-trigram bottle, and chrysanthemum paintings by Zhu Kongyang.

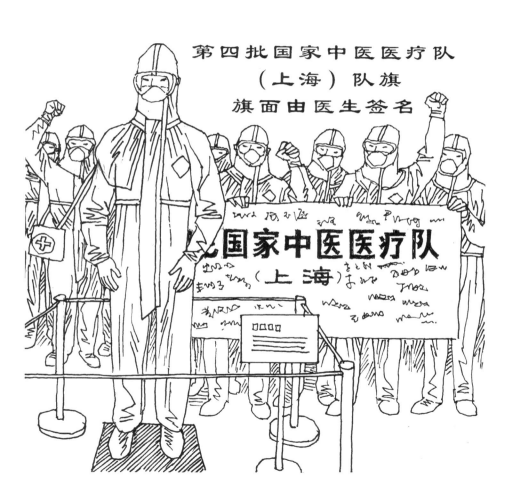